WORK.
MAMA.
LIFE.

FROM MOTHERHOOD BURNOUT
TO ABUNDANT HEALTH,
JOY AND WELLBEING

ALI YOUNG

WILEY

First published in 2022 by John Wiley & Sons Australia, Ltd

42 McDougall St, Milton Qld 4064
Office also in Melbourne

© John Wiley & Sons Australia, Ltd 2022

The moral rights of the author have been asserted.

ISBN: 978-0-730-39656-7

A catalogue record for this book is available from the National Library of Australia

Cover design by Wiley
Cover image: © Chinnapong/Shutterstock
Inside cover photo by Hayley Bracewell Photography

Disclaimer
The material in this publication is of the nature of general comment only, and does not represent professional advice. It is not intended to provide specific guidance for particular circumstances and it should not be relied on as the basis for any decision to take action or not take action on any matter which it covers. Readers should obtain professional advice where appropriate, before making any such decision. To the maximum extent permitted by law, the author and publisher disclaim all responsibility and liability to any person, arising directly or indirectly from any person taking or not taking action based on the information in this publication.

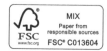

For my children, Matilda and George for gifting me motherhood, and to Pedro for supporting me on this wild soul ride I'm on.

CONTENTS

ABOUT THE AUTHOR

Dr Ali Young is a chiropractor on a mission to help mums reclaim and reset their health and their life. To rediscover their joy, self and health. After opening a private practice in Perth, Western Australia, in 2003, she soon began to work with many mums and children.

She went on to complete her Masters Level Paediatrics degree in addition to her Chiropractic degree, and through this avenue of working with more and more children, she also began to work with more and more mothers. It became highly apparent to Ali that the stress load of life could easily negatively impact not just their health but also the mums' and families' enjoyment of life.

Dr Ali became a mother for the first time herself in 2012, and with her husband moved to Malaysia as an expat mum in a foreign land. This radical shift from a very busy business owner to a mother with a minimal support group really highlighted the importance of understanding the motherhood journey, matrescence and the power of intuitive self and education.

After several moves, time as a SAHM (stay at home mum) and a FIFO (fly-in fly-out) wife/mum, and throwing one more child into the mix, her family ended up living in South Korea for two years. This is where the concept of an online community for mothers was born.

Combining her love of all things neurology, research, stress and chiropractic with her personal motherhood journey, Dr Ali created an online community, resource hub and courses for mothers the world over called UnFcK Motherhood. She continues her private practice in regional Queensland, having worked with thousands of mothers in her 20 or so years of clinical experience. She is passionate about providing mums with the opportunity to regain their health, their joy and their sense of self within their motherhood journey.

Dr Ali lives in a small seaside town on the east coast of Australia, six hours north of her closest capital city. From here, she aspires to continue empowering mothers the world over with knowledge, evidence and intuitive practices.

ACKNOWLEDGEMENTS

This book has been sitting in my brain for years, and there are a few key people who have challenged me, supported me and nurtured me to help bring her to life. I wouldn't have had my own mothering journey without the experience I had as a child with my own mum, and my two grandmothers. Growing up surrounded by so many strong (some might say stubborn ;)) women was such a blessing. My mum showed me how working mum life can be, both the good and the bad, and began to open my eyes to the possibilities. Thanks to you and Dad for your never-ending support of your crazy daughter, and to my brother for keeping me level. Nothing without Fambam.

To my soul-sister Olivia, who I owned my first practice with and who blessed me to be embraced as close as one can with her crazy triplets journey. You've been my supporter since I met you in 2003. Thanks for being my sounding board, my level head, my chiro-queen and my gin-buddy.

To the calm mums in my world. You don't know how much you show up for me, and how much you show me how to choose calm in my mothering choices. To my SIL Michelle, with your grace and composure, you show me how to be me and not lose myself. To Court, if I didn't have my dose of Calm-Court each week I think I'd be a basket case by now, and to Michelle S – the way you navigate your mothering journey is so inspiring to me, thanks for letting me in!

To the women over the years who have shaped me on my feminist ideals. From railing against early injustices with Amanda and Suemaree, to chiro discoveries with Sare, Hails, Vikkie and Laura, to the Perth Fun Days with Alicia, Joce, PD, Spag, Davi, and the Freo Crew, and to my CQ queens who listen to my babble, Jo, Hails, Em, Cass, Em, Ange, Alana and Jode. You've all been part of my mother journey.

To my team in my practice, for putting up with my big ideas with minimal follow through – thanks for keeping me ticking along through 2021. Anna – my right hand woman, thanks so much. Court – your fresh air and vibe is just what we needed and Kate, thanks for making the trek to central Queensland so I could fulfil this dream, and hopefully you can fulfil yours.

To the expat mamas who supported me in both Malaysia/Singapore and South Korea: Samira, Angela and KK, Tam, Leah, Jenn, Caz, Michelle, Yols, Anita, Sim, Nadine, Coley, and Mel, you girls helped me have the beginnings of this flame.

This book would not of been possible without the love-story of my beautiful profession, Chiropractic. If I wasn't entrenched in the deep knowing of its philosophy, and it didn't open my eyes to the magic that lies within each of us, I'd just be another peep doing a job she didn't love. Particular mention goes to James Carter and his gang back in the 2000s, and to Brandi and Don McDonald and all of the superstars in 'The Engine', for their keen insights and eye-openings, always at times when I needed that little bit of guidance.

Thank you to the amazing Tina Tower, who pitched me to Lucy at Wiley Publishing because she knew I had a story to tell, and that there were so many mums in the world who would benefit from listening in. To all of the other women building their empires in her world, I feel lucky to be a part of it.

To Wiley for taking a chance on me, and in particular to Lucy who saw something in my passion and managed, with Leigh to bring it out onto paper. To my editor Sandra, to Chris and to all of the team, thank you.

To the loves of my life — my own little fambam. For Pete for putting up with the late nights, the rants about how the world is skewed against women, how we need to do better for our kids, and still finding a way to love me. Ditto. And to my beautiful children. You gave me the gift of being a mother. You amaze me often, I love you both so much. Thanks for choosing us as your parents.

And finally, to all of the mums who have crossed my path in practice in my nearly 20 years. Each of your stories, your wins, your struggles, those tears of joy and happiness, and the ones of sorrow and sadness. This book is for you. My love story to say thank you. You have inspired me, and now it's my turn to pass the baton on. We are warrior women, we are strong. Let's lean in. Together.

INTRODUCTION

Welcome to the amazing awesomeness of motherhood!

This book is a happy by-product of my work with mums really taking off in the world. As a chiropractor, I was hands-on with mums all the time, supporting them and their kids and trying to figure out why there is so much stress in our mama world these days. So I branched into the online course world to support more mums than the ones existing in my orbit.

The real, deep-down reason, though, is that I had just escaped from a burnout myself.

I've lived it.

I've had the health challenges from it.

I know there are better ways to look after myself.

I mean, if a health-conscious health practitioner can end up in burnout, then what hope does a mama without a health background but with the same work–life balance and stress concerns have?

Crawling out of that place was pretty hard work, and looking back, I totally did it the hard way. On reflection, that is not what I want for the mums in my world. This book is kinda like my recovery love story for you, Mama. It can help you rediscover your health in some pretty easy steps; it can guide you on shifting if you want it; and my biggest aim is to give you so much info that you don't go there in the first place. This book is exactly what I wish I had been told when I was a mum in the early stages, navigating my return to work and my value as a human.

I am so excited that you've picked up this book, or been gifted it. I'm pumped that it has somehow made its way into your orbit. If this is your first lap around this motherhood game, welcome and buckle up. The adventure is phenomenal—at times tough, and at times easy. I still love it to this day! If you are a returning mama-bear, welcome back to the fray! I can't wait to help you navigate, grow and thrive through this round of your motherhood journey.

The big shift into work-life and mum-life, when and if it happens for you, is a modern ideal that is now the norm for mums and we individually navigate it in the best way possible. Thriving through this time in our life is transformative in one way, and really bloody hard in another. Escaping all the burnout challenges occurring in the world in our rushed and busy society, with the lurking pandemic hanging on, is exactly why I'm here on this earth: to help mums reconnect to their health and their 'self', and to find that spark and joy. To connect their health and their heart on this motherhood journey.

Motherhood is many things rolled into one. It's the chaos and the calm, the joy and the frustration, the overwhelm and the total fun! It's the love that you can't fathom for these little beings, who can become all encompassing. But a love that is also 100 per cent too much at times. A love that is expected to fall out of the sky the second your child is born, which happens for some, but that also takes time to build and grow for many.

For some, motherhood is a welcome interlude in a busy life, something that has been hoped and dreamed about for years. A pause in a career trajectory, a family situation or a planned event that has finally come to fruition. Our motherhood can spin in so many ways. Perhaps it will be a new beginning as you traverse back into a workplace, or working from home, or whatever the computation of working motherhood is for you.

For others, it may be more of a surprise. Maybe not planned but not unwanted. Or maybe initially it was such a shock that all the choices ran through your head to explore. Whether it's a surprise pregnancy and motherhood journey, or the whole experience of becoming a mother is nothing like the picture it's been painted as—it's a massive shift.

This shift is called 'matrescence': the glorious shift from a woman to a mother. Matrescence is going to be explored thoroughly in this book, but in these beginning stages of motherhood, I just want you to know that you aren't alone, that this is you shifting into a new version of yourself.

Working with mums so intently over the past 20-odd years from pre-conception, through matrescence and into motherhood, and especially working with their kids, I've discovered many common themes around support, annoyances, grievances and knowledge blocks that mums would like true and current info about. And there are a whole lot of ways to help a mama out.

The busy and tumultuous times that we live in require us as mothers to navigate a stress load that is quite extreme. The stress of navigating life with work (I'm a strong advocate that mothering is work, by the way, just FYI), kids, partners and expectations of society can really drive a heightened stress level in an entire household.

In this book I will share some research with you, so if you are the kind of mama who likes to know about things, you should find a lot of direction here. Like the info published in *Nature Journal* in 2019 by Azhari and others, which outlines that there is an interplay between the level of stress in parents and the synchronicity of the mother–child brain connection. Basically, this means that if the mother is stressed, there is less co-regulation (awareness of behaviours, physiological states, etc.) between mother and child—that is, they become less of a unit and the relationship suffers.

I don't know about you, but when I was hurtling towards my burnout time I was not co-regulating how I wanted to. And it felt terrible. If I can just help one mama to avoid that time in their life, or teach them how to dig themselves out when they get there, then that is a massive win for the world.

The essence of this book is about empowering mums the world over to navigate the increasing stress loads of society, particularly as working mums. And to do it with a bit more calm and quiet, health and choices during the busyness and the rush. We are going to explore our often ingrained intergenerational mothering patterns and figure out together how we can change, shift and create a new normal for us and our families.

We will be reimagining a thriving motherhood away from burnout for all mums experiencing the constant heightened stress load of life, towards a collective exploration of options to navigate a different path—to a truly connected, calm and conscious motherhood, with our health, and that of our families', intact.

I can't wait to go on this journey with you!.

About this book

This book might be set up a bit differently from what you expect. I've popped it into three core sections so you can flip around if you want, or just dive into the whole thing from the start. The whole book is designed to give you a guideline to shift and change minus the overwhelm. Small things, over time, will add up to a massive change in your world. The possibilities are exciting.

I have separated this book into three parts:

- Part I—WORK—forms the backbone of knowledge about who we are as mums. It covers the stuff that helps us know why we want to change and reflects on where we have come from. It's all about motherhood, stress, burnout, research and how society has aided and abetted us to end up where we are. This part isn't a 'how-to' guide; it's more about *what*. It's about what the hell has happened to us as a mothering culture, and in what ways can we reclaim our 'self', our spark and our heart.

- Part II—MAMA—is the *doing* section. Here, I introduce you to the 5 Pillars of Healthy Motherhood: five simple approaches you can use to create shift and change in your world. Each chapter in part II gives you heaps of tools to move yourself back into the zone of health. To explore who you are as a woman and a mother at the same time. And how they are connected and not. How time can be reclaimed so you can do it all without adding to the stress load. Ain't nobody want that!

- Part III—LIFE—is where we look at life through the lens of mother, business owner, employee, staying at home and the navigation of each of these things. We integrate these joyfully and vitally into your world using a framework that I call the 'transformation pyramid'. I'll talk about your strength of purpose, your sense of self, why *you* matter and how the way you see yourself can be life changing. Together we'll look at transformation and the lightness it can bring back into your world. By the end of part III you'll have your specific revolution plan ready to go. I can't wait to hear all your stories of shift and change!

Like I said at the start of the book, it's all about you: taking what you want and choosing your own adventure. My hope is that by the end of part III you will have found even just one new way to choose your outcomes, create connection back in your day and love yourself endlessly as a mum.

Throughout the book you will find glorious interludes. I've called them 'Pause moments'. These give you a moment to reflect and think about what you've just read. Maybe it's big for you, maybe it's a blip or maybe it's not significant at all. There is no right or wrong on this spectacular journey.

Motherhood is amazing. Working motherhood can really give us the best of both worlds. We can fill our cup for ourselves and our cup for our families, making this intentional shift with beautiful intentions, knowledge, tools and skills to make it thriving, vital and joyful!

It makes me jump whenever I read that: a world full of mums expressing their own awesome selves is my kind of nirvana. Let's get into it!

Part I
WORK (AND YOU)

Balancing Motherhood and Life

Let's explore the world of motherhood!

As I said in the introduction, this part of the book is all about arming you with the knowledge to make thoughtful and considered decisions and to be able to change when you need to. To soulfully lead your life with heart and health firmly in your grasp.

When I began the journey back to working-mum land, I knew all the right things to do ... or so I thought. I was busy, I was rushing, I was yelling ... I was trying to do it all. In this part of the book I share a lot about my motherhood journey.

I'd like to start by planting some seeds of hope that you aren't alone and that you are in the right space to learn about motherhood.

In part I we'll be looking into the knowledge and backstory of motherhood. In each chapter, I'll give you some gentle run-throughs of important stuff that will help you rediscover your awesome self and your health, and to find a bit more joy. I'll share some knowledge and research, and paint a picture of how it might show up for you. Or, at least, how I've seen it in some other mums' worlds.

I definitely had to turn on and off my researcher brain for this part of the book. My hope is that I've injected enough real life into it that you get to the end and can see the parallels in your own world. Doing the work now on the *you* part of motherhood will make understanding the *how* a lot easier.

The body is a wondrous thing. It is able to adapt and change and mould, and it responds perfectly to its environment all the time thanks to our brain and nervous system. But stress can lead us to being switched 'on' all the time, which isn't healthy. And stress is something we all had our fair share of during COVID, particularly during lockdowns. For mothers, this has had a particularly significant impact.

In this part of the book, I'll be bringing to light how your body is magical. How it's wonderful. How it's able to allow you your human existence and keep being resilient through the motherhood gig.

Enjoy learning about your awesome self because that's exactly what you are. My hope is that by the end of part I you will be able to recognise just how amazing you are and that if you're struggling a bit to balance motherhood and life (including work), you'll learn how to reclaim your 'self' again!

(1)

INTRODUCING MOTHERHOOD AND JOURNEYS

My motherhood and journeys into the great awesome unknown!

I thought I would start out on our journey of discovering burnout, mum-life, working-mum life and all the glorious in between with a bit of a discussion about my motherhood. Because sure, I can qualify myself with skills learned at uni, but there's nothing like the trenches and supporting thousands of mums along the way!

In this opening chapter you'll read a bit about:

- my motherhood journey
- burnout—how it can show up and surprise us
- support systems and stress
- patriarchy in motherhood (a quick little chat and eye opener)
- insights into healing yourself and vitality.

Observations from before I took the leap into motherhood

When I graduated from RMIT University way back in 2002, I thought motherhood was just another linear element in our life, a trajectory that a lot of women traverse along because it is the 'done' thing. As a country kid growing up in regional Victoria, I was encouraged to study one of three professions: doctor, lawyer or stockbroker. These were perceived as my way out of the country life and into a 'safe job'.

My mum worked at the hospital in town as a sonographer and I would often go there after school to wait for a lift home (town was some 45 kilometres away from our home). Interestingly, I began to observe the difficulties professional women experienced in that environment, and how they were always juggling and figuring out how to 'manage it all'.

When I was 15, I went to a chiropractor for the first time and, as well as getting rid of the pain I'd been experiencing in my feet for a long time, I learned that they could choose their own working hours. Subconsciously, choosing chiropractic — a career that is supportive of working mums — was a no-brainer. Not only had it been modelled to me as an easy working-mum choice but having been around inter-generational models of working mothers, I guess I felt well placed to 'have it all'.

As a 23-year-old chiropractor, I gave it little regard, however, and began on my lightning-fast career trajectory. This took me to the other side of Australia, all the way to Perth, where I met some amazing women who have influenced my motherhood. Love stories abound about how we all met... but I'll save that for another time!

At university, when I was studying chiropractic, there was zero focus on matrescence (the beautiful shift and change from woman to mother, something I'll be discussing in depth in chapter 3) and the stages of motherhood. We were taught about the pregnant mother, but not how to care for the post-partum one. We were taught about newborn babies, infants and toddlers. We were taught about the hormonal flux of adolescence. There was no highlight reel of the elements of motherhood we needed to be supportive of. It was pretty much glossed over. This really needs to change if we are going to support mothers in the way they need us to.

When I began practising, I was blessed to take over a private family practice and I began working closely with mums, both for themselves and as parents of the children under my care. It was here that I witnessed, firsthand, the desire of mothers to have all of the best things for their children, including health.

Mums would constantly chase the to-do list that helped them to keep their child/ren healthy, with a complete disregard for their own health. There was so much focus on doing everything for their family that stopping to care for themselves was never a priority that made it onto the completed to-do list.

This pattern would keep occurring until they fell in a heap, which is where I would step in as part of the team putting them back together.

Sound familiar? I'm sure it does for some of you. And probably not for others.

Interestingly, this was modelled to me in practice as the norm for all mums. It took until I became a mother, and explored how I could maintain my own personal vitality, to dig into these concepts of health for mums. The dichotomy of not being selfish, but choosing to care for myself as well as my child — which may be different from the expected norm in standard Western society — was a hard pill to swallow. The true expression of both mum-guilt and the 'perfect mother' myth had ingrained themselves in my thoughts around what a mother was, and it began to impact my motherhood.

I'd seen my business partner and best friend traverse a multiple pregnancy, and how the system had expectations of her to birth a certain way because she was having triplets. She sought out health professionals who supported her choice to have a vaginal birth, which somewhat made her an outlier. This then formed an element of minority fatigue throughout her mothering journey. Add to this the expectation that, because she became a mum to three amazing little humans, she was supposed to constantly be equally fully fatigued and extremely grateful.

She, however, chose something different for herself and her family. For her, work was a large part of her values system and it allowed her to feel herself amid the chaos of three tiny humans. This modelled to me the 'anti-perfect mother' myth. There were times, of course, where the mum-guilt associated with any and all decisions around return to work — or not performing at work after the kids had been up at night and she hadn't slept well — was very real. The reality of the stress of trying to maintain a perfect work–life–mum balance was extraordinary, and this was well before the crazy times of the 2020s.

‖ PAUSE MOMENT

- Did you observe friends/family/colleagues before you became a mum, who in retrospect shaped your thoughts on mothering and motherhood?
- What pre-framed ideas (like fatigue, tiredness, joy, playfulness, connection, isolation) did you take into motherhood?

My journey into motherhood

My journey into motherhood was an unplanned but much-longed-for surprise. A wedding night baby, in fact. I know...totally ironic for the health professional to have that happen, but hey, apparently it's a thing. Leading up to motherhood, I sold my practice of eight years to my best friend, got married (and pregnant) and shortly afterwards my husband and I moved to Malaysia for a work opportunity for him.

Massive life change. I was exceptionally grateful for the opportunities it offered, but it was a turbulent time too.

We moved to Johor Bahru just after my 20-week scan, with everyone telling me how lucky I was to be gifted all of this time off before the baby came to prepare for their imminent arrival. Even though I'd spent the preceding 12 years working with mums, in retrospect my preparation was, ironically, not exactly what I needed. I was highly focused on the birth and trying to dispel ingrained beliefs that I couldn't birth vaginally due to an off-the-cuff comment from a radiologist who had looked at my spine films when I was 15.

As you can imagine, being hyper-aware of the role that our inner-language can play in our birthing outcomes, I was genuinely focused on shifting that. I worked with a hypnobirthing instructor and a doula, and when I was in Australia, chatted to the midwives and an OB, relaying my fears and concerns, and acknowledging the place I was coming from prior to my baby's birth.

Needless to say, the concept of motherhood at the other side of the birth didn't really cross my mind. Not even once did we have a conversation as a couple or even within my inner circle of what to expect in my motherhood journey. I find it so interesting that I seriously spent more time worrying about the pram I chose than I did about how to parent and mother once our babe was born.

I know I'm not alone in this. On reflection, and chatting with thousands of mums since, this isn't a solo story. Many mums out there definitely go in with a similar thought construct: if I birth this babe a certain way, then all will be perfect.

This strongly feeds into the 'perfect mother' myth.

My journey into motherhood was definitely not what I expected. I travelled from Malaysia back to Perth by myself at 35+6 weeks — that is, one day before I would no longer have been allowed to fly because of the gestation of my pregnancy. I left my husband behind in Malaysia, and had three weeks by myself. The fear of going into labour and him not being able to get there in time was big. I'm sure that this led to a heightened stress response on my way into the birthing experience, and possibly the outcomes of birth too.

My birthing began with a hind water leak (a small water leak, not a massive gush) at 40+5 (so 5 days over the expected due date) that went on for a few days. I was in and out of the birthing centre for check-ups over those days. I was trying my hardest with everything to avoid an induction as I understood so intently the cascade of intervention that can happen after that time.

Nevertheless, I ended up being induced, and having a long labour. My doula was present, and every time she left the room to move her car (it went for 18 hours), someone would come in and check me. All the pressures of time were placed on me, and the experience was pretty much the complete opposite of what I had envisaged. While I ultimately avoided a caesarean, the trauma, the use of forceps and ending up in a stark theatre prepped for a caesarean really impacted my initial bonding with my child.

As soon as she was placed on my chest, I felt appreciation for her safe arrival. I felt an element of love, but I didn't feel that overwhelming, life-changing 'kapow' moment that everyone told me I would. I had super protective instincts around my child, yet I didn't feel the love-bubble gush I expected. This alone was enough to start my mum-guilt journey. At the time, I didn't realise I didn't have it, but on consideration, my love grew and grew rather than rushing in.

Over the next couple of weeks, we packed up our house in Perth so we could rent it out when we repatriated overseas again, navigated new parenthood, had both sets of parents visit from interstate, celebrated Christmas and then flew back to Malaysia with a 20-day-old child. It felt 'normal' at the time, but on reflection it was pretty bloody crazy.

No wonder I felt a little lost.

To top it off, I had all my people trying to help me with advice on what they perceived was or wasn't working with my newborn.

Have you heard these ones?

- Why is she feeding so much?
- Why is feeding taking so long?
- Why is she so small?
- You should be doing ...
- You shouldn't be doing ...
- You do this with a nappy ...
- You do this other thing with a dummy ...
- You wrap her this or that way ...

I was thrust into discovering that my own personal, good-enough mother concept was based on external elements of the newborn phase like sleep, poo, feeding and settledness. And I pretty much felt like a bit of a failure because, while for years I'd been able to support mothers with the health of their kids, my own child didn't fit the perfect 'box' of what a 'good' baby does. This common societal measure of a good mother being reliant upon how her child shows up for certain benchmarks really fuelled my unhappiness at the time.

Moving back to Malaysia was isolating. Comparatively, I imagine it was a little like birthing during lockdown and remaining home all the time, with minimal community connection and support being offered. I haven't had to live through significant lockdown in Australia, but in conversation and while supporting women who have, it feels like I had the same brain-based trauma response they experienced. I began doing the things that I thought good mothers did. I exercised, I cooked, I responded to my child as she needed and I 'wifed' like a champion.

And yet, I felt like I wasn't a good mother because my daughter thought sleep was for the weak. There wasn't a sleep book I didn't read, there wasn't a friend I didn't lean into, there wasn't advice I didn't think to add to my daily 'should-do'. But not much helped. Ironically.

And yet, here I am, writing a book on supporting mums to choose their own adventure. I am so thankful for the crazy early introduction to motherhood, as it certainly shaped my journey, my learnings and my passion for mums.

Support systems and stress

While my support systems were there, I was creating stress for myself and within my family because I was striving to fill a 'perfect child and perfect mother' ideology. It wasn't a conscious thing. I just did it because that's what I thought I was supposed to do. I know I'm not alone here. It's well researched. It's the intensive mothering ideology that we will explore as we move through this book, and how it impacts the stress load of mothering. This ideology is creating a cycle of burned-out working mums trying to do and be all to everyone, except for themselves. A bit more on that soon.

Moving through this as an individual, and reflecting on it over the years since my first child was born, highlights to me how, even as a highly knowledgeable mother, this matrescence period can really impact us, our future health and the lens through which we view motherhood.

As a mum, the stress load of life external to our 'self', and internal within our specific environment can impact us so innately that it alters our health, our vitality, our zest and, ultimately, our mothering. The amazing support systems we are gifted by our Western culture can be lifechanging. They can literally turn a really crappy, depressive and anxious experience into something joyful and vital.

The support systems offered to mothers, as reported anecdotally in my practice, have at times been overwhelming, and 'too much'. As mums have told me, there can be conflicting advice, given within short time frames, that can raise anxiety levels. And when mothers look externally to find all of the answers, it can also be a hugely overwhelming experience. Instead, giving ourselves permission to listen within, to listen to our calm and that inner voice, can allow us to support ourselves in a way that suits us.

The level of stress that comes from a lack of our own knowledge and because we continually have to source information from external sources can be the first step towards burnout in my experience. When we then add in mum-guilt and returning to work, it's a recipe for disaster.

NEWBORN PHASE OF MOTHERING

+

SUPPORT SYSTEM STRESS

+

STRONG EXTERNAL INFLUENCES

= A PRIME RECIPE FOR BURNOUT!

Unsurprisingly, my daughter Matilda one day began to sleep, and we then decided to jump on the child number two rollercoaster. I mean, of course we did, ha ha. This journey was completely different and I often reflect on my second birth as being my healing delivery. No intervention, the instant love was there and the shift to a family with two children was a wholly different experience.

And while this was a healing birth, it didn't mean that I didn't get stressed ... that I didn't search outside of me for answers on how things were going and what I should be doing. It just meant I began with a little bit of a head start on the time before.

‖ PAUSE MOMENT

- I viewed my second birth as a 'healing birth', making up for the first one. Did you do that too?
- Learning to listen to my gut instinct took time and patience. The first time it was about deciding not to use controlled crying. Do you listen to your gut instinct?

From burnout to vitality

The burnout in my world didn't happen until well after the newborn years. I had returned to work, opened a practice, traversed difficulty navigating a 'normal life' back in Australia ... and some familial stress was thrown in for good measure.

It was a recipe for burnout. It kinda crept up on me, and had to yell at me to really get my attention. It actually happened prior to COVID, and it just kinda got a kick along and continued when that whole debacle happened.

Lockdown life, particularly in Australia, is a recipe for neurological burnout. Healing from it, and learning how to regain my joy, fun, vitality and health was amazing. And this journey from burnout to vitality is what this book is all about.

Each foray into motherhood comes with its own challenges and wins. It presents opportunities for growth and expansion, discovery and a sense of awakening and reflection for yourself. This reflection on my own journey, the re-introduction of mountains of neurological reading and information about motherhood, the child–mother relationship, how our brains function, and the impact of stress, burnout and a COVID-impacted society on our health and our 'self' led me down the rabbit hole of a thriving motherhood.

I can't wait to explore this with you.

(2)

A MOTHERHOOD OF EXPECTATIONS

How the stories we tell ourselves can make or break our experience!

I remember when I was a first-time mum, I felt the weight of expectation on my shoulders hard. I was in a foreign country with a three week old, an apartment, no car and a husband at work all day. In my mind, I was expected to keep the baby alive, to keep everything clean, to make nourishing food. I mean, man! How about you?

I also felt extreme joy and gratitude that there was this little person hanging out with me all day. I mean, she was cute and stuff. She did poo, wee, she boobed, she slept occasionally. *Joy!*

I craved the joy and the togetherness with her ... and yet there was a niggle in the back of my mind. I felt a niggle to begin to look a certain way, to exercise, to not get too upset, to be in control, to never feel guilty or burned out or tired, to have my child 'behave' in a certain way. My perception was that my mothering was predicated by how well she did certain things.

This chapter is probably a little heavy on the concepts of society and motherhood. But remember that part I of the book is giving you the background to step into your awesome health and vitality with all the knowledge you need.

In this chapter we are going to explore:

- our inner critic as a mother—you know, that mean girl inside our mind!
- intergenerational motherhood: how the way we were mothered impacts our mothering
- the five common societal expectations of motherhood
- a quick expectation shake-off method.

Commonly, we poor mums have a lot of questions shoved in our general direction. I mean, really, do we want to judge our mothering on things that we have minimal control over?

- Is she sleeping well?

- Are you getting enough sleep?

- Have you read this book or that book?

- Are you following what this person has told you?

- Are they the right expert to be following?

- Are they the ones who are going to give you the best information?

Feeling all the expectations to wade through the information out there and derive the most knowledge out of the available resources and then put it to good use was a thing (a thing that I very much didn't enjoy!). As a professional woman, and particularly one in the health sector, I was supposed to do this better than the woman who didn't fit into this demographic of mother.

As a health professional who worked with babies and mums for a living, I felt that I couldn't ever fail. Failure meant, in my mind, that I was not a good health professional. The mothering I was doing was commentary on my 'fitness' to be a health professional. The internal judging if I felt I wasn't doing a great job. And when I chose to go back to work, how could anybody trust me again because I clearly sucked at this motherhood gig when it came to living it myself. So let's dive into how I fell into the society trap, and how I can help you get out of it a little easier using some simple steps.

Our inner critic: that mean girl mum living inside of us

Have you ever watched the movie *Mean Girls*? I love that film. I mean, of course I was not a mean girl. At least not to others ... but most definitely to myself at times.

Now, as a mama, I recognise a little bit of mean girl lives in my brain. You know, that mean girl telling you that you should have done something a different way. You should have:

- had a different conversation about disappointment with your child
- taken time off to go to the swimming carnival at school
- not taken time off to go to the swimming carnival coz, you know, profit and loss statements are a thing to consider
- not booked that massage
- gone for a run —*fatty!*
- not gone for a run — kid time is more important.

That bloody mean girl has a lot to answer for, right?

Your narrative is probably quite different from mine. I mean, our mean girls take on a whole different voice for ourselves. Maybe your inner critic said differing things to you. But the one thing that drives all of our inner critics are *expectations*.

In the previous chapter we explored some of the elements that drive our mothering experience. In this chapter, let's have a look at these expectations as they play out in the motherhood world, with a lens specifically focused on us as mothers.

Before we step into this in the motherhood sphere, having a basic understanding of the psychology of the inner critic (mean girl), inner voice (awesome girl) and expectations (noisy world) provides a great basis for the understanding of how this fits in. In a comprehensively researched article on the website Positive Psychology, professor of cultural history at the University of Kent, Anna Katharina Schaffner writes about living with our inner critic. I love how she has condensed our understanding of this into automatic negative thoughts (ANTs), also commonly called negative self-talk. I just like to call it my mean girl! Go to the resources at the back of this book for info on her article.

Our mean girl is established in our childhood, and she basically materialises when we begin to look at common things in our environment through the lens of 'the way we should do things'. This means she creates ideal scenarios in our mind of things we should do and say — things that may be beyond our capability at the time so we tend to fall short. This mean girl voice is there to act as a bit of a protector in our brain function. Seems weird, I know, but basically, if this voice perceives danger, which is something outside of 'the way we should do things', she fires off our fright/flight responses.

This mean girl exists as a psychological protective mechanism to give us a sense of what is occurring in our environment, to allow this fright/flight response to function well. According to Schaffner, it can show up internally if, when we were children, we felt unloved or constantly criticised and we blamed ourselves rather than our parents (total mean girl moment), creating a survival mechanism to dampen this reflex.

Schaffner says the best way to get rid of those recurrent mean girl moments is to change your narrative. This just means, when you hear yourself criticising the things you are doing, do these three things:

1. Recognise that it's a mean girl moment. Feel the response in your body when it's there.

2. Think about what you would rather say to yourself (imagine you are your best mate).

3. Rinse and repeat. One sure way to get rid of that mean girl voice is to constantly shut her up and change what she says.

How does this play out in a real-world setting? Let's look at it simply in mum terms. Imagine that your babe can't string those 'important' sleep cycles together. So they are only sleeping for 20- to 40-minute windows. That's a mean girl mum fail right there.

What that mean girl voice is doing, is increasing your stress response by making you constantly feel like you've failed. Over time, that ramps up your stress load and can create a more stressful mothering experience.

No thanks. I don't see that for you. I lived it for me. It ain't great.

Let's kick our mean girls to the curb!

The expectations and stories that are peddled in society as the norm are driving an alteration in our mean girl inner critic, and they can stop us from exploring the realities of what motherhood and our expectations of it truly are.

The mothering conundrum of expectation I feel is twofold. But before I jump into that, let's take a moment to pause together.

‖ PAUSE MOMENT

- Who's your mean girl in your head? Is she a Heather? A Courtney? Is she a Disney Princess turned bad? Or just you, in a different form?

- Is there something she keeps saying that you know isn't true?

- What do you wish came out of your mean girl's mouth?

Intergenerational mothering: how our mothering is passed along

Expectations can play a large part in mothering. We've kind of established that now. It would be remiss of me to not have a chat about how the generations of mothering that we observe impact how we mother. According to the Center on the Developing Child at Harvard University, our brain lays down the majority of its circuits and pathways in the first few years of life (up until six to seven years of age). My theory is that we learn how to mother from how we are mothered in those first few years. I mean, have you ever listened to yourself and thought, *Holy shit — I sound exactly like my mum!*

I often wonder how these early years nurturing moments that we experience as a child play out in the subconscious roll-out of our own mothering? How do we take them on board and create our level of expectation of our own mothering?

Researchers such as Madden and associates call this theory 'intergenerational parenting'. They look at how our own maternal mothering can play out in the way we express our mothering habits. In their excellent study, they found that the parenting ideals shown by grandmothers are associated with the parenting actions of both the mothers and the fathers. Basically, this tells us that how we choose to show up for our kids could be of benefit for their children in the future. That's pretty epic — and also a little bit stressful, particularly when your mean girl is telling you that you are *not* doing a great job. This is where knowledge doesn't always bring freedom. If we are experiencing anxieties around 'how good we are' and the 'good enough mother' phenomenon, this knowledge can bring some relief as to why you do things in such an ingrained and certain way.

However, shifting this lens a little, we can see how the role that our predecessors in this parenting gig played could genetically and sociologically impact the things we believe, the structures we choose to bring to our mothering and the way we can make it work. At the very least, we can perhaps see where our mean girl voice might come from sometimes, an expectation that has shown up from early nurturing.

One of my dearest girlfriends reflects on this quite often. She is the mother to two young kids (at the time of writing), and she had to wade through many years of infertility to get her kids. Through this, she developed strong expectations that she would not be the martyr mother (the mother who gives everything to their kids, leaving nothing in the tank) and would be a 'good mum' — because she knew she wanted something different for her own mothering compared to how her mum mothered her. Her kids were really hard to come by, so to be the best mother that she could possibly be for her much desired family she had to be true to herself!

Throughout her childhood, her mum made a big deal of being the martyr, of doing everything for her kids. And, as they got older, of letting them know about it too. She showed up as the mum who gave up her everything for them. As my girlfriend began her mothering journey as an older mum with a career to boot, she was highly aware of this story and worked hard at honouring herself and not letting go of who she was. It could have been easy for her to slip into martyr mode — but she knew that wasn't what she wanted.

She did this because this was the model she was shown and she didn't want it. Being aware enough to honour herself, her own desires and who she needed to be, and to show up as the mother she wanted to be, was such beautiful mothering to witness.

II PAUSE MOMENT

- Have you ever thought about how you were 'mothered'?
- Do you catch yourself sounding like your mum, or grandma or significant caregiver?
- Is there any one thing you do that your mum did that you wish you could stop? (Mine is banshee yelling that dinner is ready while the kids are outside—OMG, such a trigger).

The 5 common societal expectations of mothering

Societal expectations can sometimes be the heaviest kind of expectations in mothering. I don't want that for you. I just want to give you a bit of an overview as to how you can be shaped to do things a certain way without even realising it. Society can create a massive load of life on mothers, especially those of us who work and mother together.

I'm going to break this down into five easy-to-handle ideas. Take them or leave them as you will.

I always had an inkling of them, but when I worked with the amazing motherhood studies sociologist Dr Sophie Brock — with whom I completed a motherhood practitioner certification — she opened my eyes about how it really unfolds for heaps of mums out there. I found just being gifted the basics of understanding behind all of this was enough for me to personally change and recognise things I wanted to alter in my mothering. Ultimately, it was to bring down the stress load, and up the joy mode. My hope is that something in these five concepts brings you a little 'aha' moment too. These small 'aha' moments can build up to magic change.

With your permission, let us begin!

(1) Mothers should behave a certain way

As you can probably imagine, with an online platform called UnFcK Motherhood, this one really gets my goat. The societal expectations that mothers should conform to a mothering norm or standard in their behaviours is pervasive. As women in an industrialised Western world, we are often encouraged to explore our sense of self and being in a whole-woman construct. Shouldn't that mean that we are free to figure out who the hell we are? Yet, as soon as we become mums, there's a bit less of that freedom in the figuring out.

As mums, there are perceptions around our calmness, our quietness and what nurturing should look like. We are supposed to fit a certain mould of normal and good mothering. We are encouraged to behave as if we didn't have a separate life before that is worthy of continuing on with. The measure of being a great mum is to not grieve what you have stopped doing, but to only *love* all this newness in your world.

Do you remember that song from the 90s 'Don't Worry, Be Happy' (pick the lass who was a teen then)? It's this kind of toxic positivity that we are expected to adopt in motherhood. When we throw working-mum life on top of this behaviour expectation, we are suddenly thrust into a world that might not suit us.

We can choose our own story. Take me, for example. I had a pretty fun youth and loved a lot of loud music, dancing and socialisation. Yet as a mother, if I put on my favourite 90s Seattle grunge band, danced in my kitchen and wanted to take my kids for a lunch at the pub with my girlfriends, there might just be some questions from well-meaning people. Probably from people I might not bother about (jokes, sort of), but it is outside the norm to do these activities with the kids regularly.

Our behaviours, as long as they are safe for us and our children, are just that: our behaviours. My nurturing style is highly different from that of many of the mums who come through my practice doors. Yet I know that I have a great bond with my kids, that our mother–child love is there. They don't care that their mum has crazy hair and dances around to silly music (as long as none of their friends are there to watch anyway — coz that is soooo embarrassing) and I'm proud that I've introduced them to things I loved like Pearl Jam and Masters at Work ... because these stories and bands have shaped me.

The expectation of putting ourselves aside for the perceived benefit of our children is driving a decline in the joy of motherhood.

There. I said it. We need to honour ourselves and who we are to allow our mothering and motherhood to be easy, calm and connected.

(2) Mothers should look a certain way

Ah ... the pre-baby body phenomenon. Does it make your skin crawl too? The push of mothers to achieve their pre-baby bodies is well understood. In a 2004 article, Professors Shari Dworkin and Faye Wachs dived into the phenomenon of how past feminist uprisings have been used to create the link between looking 'great' and our ability to mother well. I mean seriously, WTAF?

One of the key points in this article that really clarifies the outside-in view of the female body is: 'Exactly at the moment when a woman's body is accomplishing a highly valued route to femininity, she is least likely to be viewed as aesthetically ideal'. It's the view that while pregnancy is a great thing, it isn't an attractive thing. In my experience, other females notice how we are 'looking great and glowing' through our pregnancies. Yet there are perceived responsibilities that once we have a child, we will go back to looking and being exactly as we were before.

A survey conducted online by BabyCenter of 7000 new mothers identified some key points in the after-baby-body world. It found that 64 per cent of the survey takers felt their body image had gotten worse after they became a mother. Interestingly, it also found that over time, even if mums lost the weight, their body image remained altered in 62 per cent of the population. That's a lot of body image concerns we are carrying around.

Mothers have enough changes in their world learning how to care for this new little person, and how to navigate a whole new existence. I mean, they've just momentously birthed, passing into matrescence and their new sense of self (more on that in the next chapter). Well done, Mama! Being concerned about getting their body back should be one of the lowest things on their agenda.

Expectations that within weeks after birth you appear as if you haven't been pregnant at all abound. If we look at the social commentary around celebrities after they've had children, you can see the continual seeding of this narrative into the psyche of mothers worldwide.

I remember when we were living in South Korea — my husband and I moved there when our kids were two and one years old — we got a group of mums together to exercise. This was a super precious time for me as I didn't know anybody and it allowed me to forge beautiful friendships. On reflection, there was definitely an undercurrent of exercising together to allow ourselves to look a certain way (and can I just say that all of us were healthy and looking after ourselves and our kids well). Many conversations were had on how to best feed ourselves without losing milk supply or energy levels to allow us to get that old body back again.

Hell, I juice-fasted, I ate a low-carb diet, I did everything to make myself look like I did before I had kids. And I never questioned it. I just thought that was what I was supposed to do. It was an expectation of my motherhood that I was a successful mother if I looked a certain way. And that was defined by my pre-baby self.

Zero recognition was given to how the process of becoming a mother changed my physical being. Zero acknowledgement for growing babies, the widening of the ribcage, the softening of pelvis shape, the years of breastfeeding.

Nope... it was all about fitting back into the dresses of years past and being happy with my sense of self, which was based on this external perception of what that was. It's time we all started calling bullshit on this. I didn't know any better... and one of my core desires is to help mums recognise they are more than just the way they look!

(3) Mothers should 'parent' a certain way

I don't want to be controversial in this land, but there are so many ways we can parent. In my experience, there most definitely isn't a right or wrong way that fits everybody, their family unit and their children. I went into this whole mothering gig with an expectation that I would parent in a very specific way, while still being unsure how to mother. I'm not sure where I grabbed the info from and what subconscious pathways it had been built through, but there were ways that I perceived to be the 'right way' to parent.

The 'right way' when I became a new mum looked completely different from how I parent now. It's an evolving thing. But interestingly, the perceived expectation of how a parent should do it is high. Research by Kate Harwood, Neil McLean and Kevin Durkin identified that those mothers who went in with an optimistic (or positive) outlook were much more likely to have matched or exceeded expectations. However, when the 'experiences were negative relative to expectations, there was greater depression symptomatology and poorer relationship adjustment'. What this means is that if you go into parenting thinking it will be great, and it is, then you have a great time. However, if you go into parenting and it isn't as good as you thought it would be, it just makes you more likely to have depression and anxiety. The perception of what parenting should be and look like can impact the mental health of our mums.

Remember back in chapter 1, where I talked about newborn times predicating burnout? This is exactly what I meant. If we can create realistic expectations of parenting, and how changing what you do is normal, then we are much less likely to end up in burnout land.

I can categorically say that I went into motherhood with pretty high expectations of glorious calm days, lots of connected play, ease with breastfeeding and sleep … you know, all the pretty pictures. Yet there are some questions that I wish I'd asked and discussed with my husband before we began the journey that could have made it a whole lot simpler.

I wish we had discussed:

- How will we share child rearing duties? How does each of us see the make-up of day and night?

- What support can we expect to have to help us achieve our parenting and family ideals?

- What religion/ethics/mindset will we aim to develop in our child/ren?

- To smack or not to smack?

- Who would ideally look after the child/ren if both parents are working?

- What would an ideal childhood look like to me now, as an adult? How can we create this for our child/ren?

- What does a happy and healthy parent look like?

- What does a happy and healthy child look like?

- Are there any cultural significances we each bring to the table? How can we incorporate those?

- How can we each connect socially to our friends and mindfully with ourselves? How can we keep our relationship alive?

Mindfulness being brought pre-emptively into the parenting journey before we embark on it is an amazing way to kick off the shackles of 'should'.

Those first six to eight weeks (or months) can be so life altering, and having a plan together (or with your support people if you are doing this gig solo) is so very important. If we can head into parenting with an open heart and mind, and decrease the 'shoulds', imagine where that can lead us.

(4) Mothers should be selfless all the time

Okay, this probably doesn't need a great deal of discussion, but the martyr or selfless mother concept is a biggie in the expectation stakes. Research conducted by Lazarus and Rossouw in 2015 discovered that it was vital to educate women about societal expectations and self-expectations prior to having a child, as 'these expectations can influence levels of self-esteem, depression, anxiety, and stress'. Much like in point 3, how we think it will end up and how it actually does can drive our mental health outcomes.

Where point 4 differs is that we are focusing not on the parenting journey, but on how your selflessness as a mother is indicative of the intensity of your love for those little babes. The self-scrutiny of failure around not being selfless is massive. There is a gap in our current health system with a lot of blame levelled at mothers, who are ultimately trying their best, if their child isn't doing things the 'normal' way. Society expects that if we are doing everything as we should, our baby will just follow along the curve.

This isn't always true. I mean, it's most definitely *not true*!

In my opinion, the martyr mother phenomenon doesn't serve anyone in the mother–child relationship. According to research by Mikolajczak and Roskam in 2020, we need a shift in focus from us as parents being responsible solely for good childhood development outcomes. I mean, the Convention of the Rights of the Child determines how our kids 'should be developing', and it even says that when we look after ourselves, ensuring our own wellbeing, it decreases parental burnout and improves development outcomes for the kiddos.

Martyrdom leads to parental exhaustion and burnout. The pandemic of 2020/22 (and hopefully no longer) exacerbated the pressure on parents to do everything for their kids so they wouldn't be damaged by the lockdown, home learning, altered social structures and the complete upheaval of life as we generally knew it. Yet, when we are busily trying to work and parent and school, putting the kids first all the time in this selfless parenting paradigm can be really damaging.

The burnout you are feeling in the life you are struggling to live is where you can begin to make shifts for your health and your 'self'. And hopefully empower those little people in your life while you're at it too!

(5) Mothers shouldn't have their own aspirations or desires for life as this makes them selfish

Okay, the last one is a biggie. I reckon it's big in my mind because it was the one I had to really overcome. Feeling selfish while also doing the things that light you up on the inside can be a really tough road to navigate. Yes, there is a shift that women matter in the workforce. The gender pay gap in Australia is slightly improved. But there aren't the supports out there to make us feel great about doing all the things that busy working mums love or need to do to make life work. I'm still not convinced that we are shifting around the fluidity of mothers' desires and career aspirations.

Let me give you an example here. My best friend, Olivia, prior to having her kids, owned and operated a multi-doctor chiropractic practice. She was the director of a franchise for other chiropractic practices also. Once she had her triplets, there was an expectation that she would just want to stay at home. It was assumed, particularly I think because she was having multiples, that there would be no role more fulfilling than that of mother in her life now.

Yet after the boys were born and the family had settled into their new life well, she had a desire to return to practice. It was her desire. Her inner sense of service. And it was frowned down on because, obviously, all she should have wanted to be was a mum. These are the kinds of societal expectations that can really impact our motherhood journey. I'm so proud of her for choosing what worked for her. For choosing to stand up for her innate knowledge and go back initially for four to five hours per week.

Her kids are now teenagers, and they most certainly didn't suffer with her going back to work. Some would say they are really balanced and have been shown that a woman can be strong and nurturing at the same time. That a mum can own a business, manage staff and be loving to her own family too.

However, if society doesn't afford us these opportunities, how are we supposed to explore ourselves, connect with our callings again, strive for our career? We aren't. And it makes us a bad mum if we even have these thoughts, especially in the early days of motherhood.

Expectation is just that. Perception of an expected or desired outcome, and it is rife in our mother world. My hope for you, as you progress through this book, is that you can throw off the shackles of expectation and explore who you are, what this means, how it looks and what is going to make you sing on the inside, in your soul, listening to your intuitive self, to thrive through your motherhood.

‖ PAUSE MOMENT

- Take a moment to reflect on these five expectations placed on mothers. Have you felt that any of these have impacted your mothering?
- How would it look if you could choose differently now?

(3)

MATRESCENCE: FROM WOMAN TO MOTHER

The journey of a baby at birth isn't just that the baby is born. It's that the woman also shifts into motherhood: the birth of a mother.

The term 'matrescence' is one I only discovered a few years ago, and it 100 per cent blew my socks off. As I began to delve into the literature — and the concept of motherhood, mothering and the shift in health that occurs when we begin to give of ourselves to others so unconsciously — this term came up time and time again. It was a lightbulb moment for me that there is a term that in its full form encompasses the shifts that occur in women when they become mothers. When we begin our motherhood journey, an unmistakable change happens innately: one that for generations had remained unnamed.

A change that unlocks something inside us that we didn't even know needed unlocking, and allows us to explore our future self as a mother.

It truly is as palpable as it is real. Matrescence, a term first coined in 1973 by anthropologist Dana Raphael, is defined by psychologist, Aurélie Athan Ph.D., of Columbia University on her website, matrescence.com, as being:

> a developmental passage where a woman transitions through pre-conception, pregnancy and birth, surrogacy or adoption, to the postnatal period and beyond. The exact length of matrescence is individual, recurs with each child, and may arguably last a lifetime!

Athan expands on this to equate the change to adolescence, noting that the shift 'encompass multiple domains — bio-psycho-social-political-spiritual'. I think this really sums up the shift beautifully. This surge in physiology, neurology and psychology allows us to change at the speed of light, just like we do as we move through adolescence.

In this chapter, we are going to explore matrescence. There is a beautiful book by journalist, researcher, author, coach and mother Amy Taylor Kabbaz, *Mama Rising*, that examines this topic. But for our purposes, we're going to stick to a few simple things that will give you the knowledge to make choices in the future, choices that work for *you*. We will examine:

- what matrescence actually is
- grieving your old life (and why that's 100 per cent normal)
- normal hormonal shifts around birth time
- mum-guilt
- the internal shift in working mums with matrescence.

I trust that by the end of the chapter you will be consciously aware of the awesome changes that happened for you internally, and that have innately shaped your journey of 'self' in the mother world!

What is matrescence?

Matrescence is a deep shift within women that we often (but not always) sense is happening when we become a mother. A rising up of a new self and a grieving of the old self. As we will explore further in the chapter, this shifting sense is often not acknowledged, and the guilt and change elements are only minimally explored, understood or supported.

The psychological shift that accompanies matrescence has had more research behind it than the physiological one. We know that psychologically there is a huge life transition from being a woman to being a mother. It all sounds easy on paper, yet there are so many factors that drive our experience of it. I mean, we've just moved from being an independent woman to having this little being (or beings) solely reliant on us for everything. It's bloody massive. Can we just take a minute to acknowledge that!

Dana Raphael, the leading anthropological researcher in this field, discusses how this shift doesn't magically end when the baby is 12 months old (which is when society generally assumes mum can go back to work, and resume her old life as if nothing has altered) but continues throughout a mother's life. It is altered with each subsequent child and I think it never really stops. It's a complex rite of passage for mothers, yet once a child is born, our role is often perceived as merely to support our child in their growth and development.

As mothers, we bring a whole host of 'before' stuff to this new adventure. On her 'More to Mum' blog, the beautiful Louise East discusses this perfectly. Louise explores concepts of bringing our old 'self' to our mothering journey, and how all the things that may have made us succeed prior to our motherhood — such as structure and drive — could just be the catalyst for tough times when we begin motherhood.

When undertaking my motherhood practitioner certification with Dr Sophie Brock, she helped me discover in depth the role and shifting perceptions of mothers through this matrescence period. This allowed me to examine the concept of matrescence and how it can alter our lives in ways such as the following:

- We create stories, dreams and expectations before we are pregnant that are added to or altered as we traverse pregnancy. These ideals come from our intergenerational programming of what is a 'good mother' and can shape our internal thoughts and thinking when we begin our mothering journey.

- What we used to discuss in our 'before baby' life is now often seen as null and void as we navigate the post-baby discussions of sleep, breastfeeding, baby activities and new 'mum friends'.

- We may have previously had a career that was important to us, and now our career is altered. Getting time off to work can be challenging and our finances can be affected accordingly. Our measure of self-worth as we have experienced it previously is perhaps also significantly different.

- We now have responsibility for keeping alive a new little human. This alone is *big*!

- The physiological changes in our hormones can create emotions we may not have had to navigate before. We often have a perception of these being wrong, when in fact they are generally normal parts of being a new mum. They can lead to feelings of worry, anxiety, disappointment, guilt, fear, anger and inadequacy.

- We may begin reflecting on how we were mothered and how this is influencing the choices we make. The awareness of intergenerational mothering and how we subconsciously take on the mothering elements of the women who came before us — and the choices we make in our own mothering and our heritage and legacy — is a large awakening for many mums.

- How we view the world, and how the world views us, is changed forever once we become mums.

- We are exposed to the 'good mother' conundrum: constantly aiming for the perfect outcome in all scenarios and the slow unravelling of this striving for perfectionism, and the shift into trusting our intuition over time to stop the bad mother vs good mother fighting.

Matrescence can be confusing, with all its shifts and alterations around who we are, what we believe and how we are viewed in the world. This shift is often ignored and largely not spoken about. Imagine the freedom we could bring each other if we were open and honest in our discussions about our experiences!

II PAUSE MOMENT

- In what area of your shift to motherhood were you most surprised by your experience and/or feelings around it?
- If you could go back in time, what would you tell yourself in preparation for the shift to motherhood?

Grieving our old life

Saying goodbye to old you as you welcome new you can be a biggie. That sense of ourselves as an individual in the world, discarded as soon as we birth a human, is something we can definitely long for. I mean, I desperately clung on to my career path in any way I could just to subconsciously reinforce that I still mattered in my world. This unacknowledged reality of transition and how it can affect so many elements of our world needs a lot more voice. Supporting mothers as they move into this new motherhood journey, and allowing them space to feel the feels, to express the emotions, to not feel bad if they are not always loving this change — this is vital.

Bringing a positivity to the grief of their old life could be the shift that allows mums to be 'in' their mothering mode at the appropriate time, and to be 'in' their working mode at the appropriate time.

In my experience, discussion often centres around the concept of shame and discrediting the feelings that the mother is experiencing. How could we be so sad at a time when we should be so full of love? How can we be grieving our old life when our new life should be filling us with such joy? How can we not know what to do when we've given birth to this child?

Yet we don't ... often.

We are scared to ask for help.

We are reeling from the huge shift of birth.

We are sore.

We are celebratory but tired at the same time.

It's only natural for us to be grieving our old lives. I mean f*ck, there are still days where I wish I could jump on my bike, ride to my mate's house and sit around and drink champagne all night without a care in the world. Or fly to that conference at the last minute because it sounds good, without having to organise a precision execution of child movements to make it happen.

It's okay to grieve that. It makes you human. The societal expectation that a mother will just snap from doing all the stuff from her old life to doing the new stuff that is nearly completely centred around this little person is significant. The undertones that you are a bad mother if you question any element of this journey are still rife. The hormonal shifts creating those emotions are perceived as weak. I mean, how often are we told that it's 'just the baby blues' and we'll get over it.

Surely in the twenty-first century we can craft better responses than this.

We need to speak up with our mum friends, discuss the missing elements. Discuss the things we believe we are missing out on. Be honest about the hard bits too. And with them, maybe we can bring in some thankfulness for just one piece of the mothering experience that is okay in that present moment. Maybe it's being thankful to have excuses for day naps. Or your newborn's head smell. Or the fact you are enjoying having a C-cup for the first time in your life (maybe that's just me ... I mean, my tiny A cups got a boost and it was great while it lasted).

I just want to jump in here though, as we get stuck into the heaviness of this concept, to acknowledge that not all mothers feel this grief. In fact, there are many out there who explore their matrescence from a completely different lens: one of joy, rejoicing and expansion.

I absolutely want to honour the fact that, as women, we can have either of these experiences. We can feel the joy, the fun and the excitement of this new life adventure ... and occasionally feel the loss too.

What we need to be mindful of is understanding that this grief is a normal component of our mothering journey, and it doesn't make us unworthy of our motherhood. If we don't acknowledge it, it can morph into anger. The anger can't be stopped through toxic positivity. We need to address this as the feeling comes up.

And don't worry, I've totally got your back. Parts II and III of the book encompass this. Together, we'll discover how to rediscover joy, how to calm ourselves out of stress and how to rediscover our connection. For now, I really want to make you aware that this shift of self is hard. It's probably designed to be hard for some reason, as mothering is separate from who you are as a mother and as a woman. Acknowledging this, especially through the lens of a working mum who goes back to a career (or not) that you may have stopped for a period of time, and the grief you may then feel about no longer being at home all the time ... oh, the struggle is real. But you're not alone.

Remember that you've created a new being, but you've also created a journey to a new you. We come in with our ideals of what this is, yet we don't know what that's going to look like. We don't know who we will become. And it can be really daunting, exciting, anxiety inducing ... all of these things.

I remember being told — either subliminally through time or directly through conversation — that there is no greater feeling than when you hold your baby for the first time. That there is a love-pop reaction that instantly makes you be a great mother and you immediately undergo an internal change. This is expected, and if it doesn't happen, then maybe you aren't fit for motherhood, or you did something wrong.

I didn't have that.

My birthing was challenging and it just didn't happen for me.

I grew into love.

I felt like a bad mother because it wasn't so straight up for me.

I'd fallen for the story.

I also have many friends for whom that did happen. And some for whom it didn't.

My village was a huge part in making me see that I wasn't going crazy.

In reflection, I know that my matrescence story is not unusual. But I felt that I was a failure. The collective of women surrounding me made it feel like I was okay, yet it took me a while to understand this. At first I didn't want to talk about my failings, but eventually I opened up.

Matrescence isn't perfect for everybody. This psychological shift into the unknown that we are expected to know is massive.

❚❚ PAUSE MOMENT

- Have you felt sad about being a mum? Or for your loss of your old life?
- What's one thing that could momentarily transport you back to your old life? For me, it's a gin and tonic and inappropriately loud dance music.

Hormonal shifts

The physiological or physical shift of motherhood can be extremely different from our expectations and outcomes in motherhood and in our sense of self. During birthing, we are exposed to four key hormone transitions which, during a normal physiological birth, can influence the post-partum and newborn periods. In a standout article, 'Executive summary of hormonal physiology of childbearing: evidence and implications for women, babies, and maternity care', Sarah Buckley explores the physiology of the hormone systems of birth, namely oxytocin, beta-endorphins, epinephrine-norepinephrine (and related stress hormones) and prolactin.

Dr Buckley identifies that physiological (meaning as it happens in your body) changes facilitates beneficial

> outcomes in women and babies by promoting fetal readiness for birth and safety during labor, enhancing labor effectiveness, providing physiological help with labor stress and pain, promoting maternal and newborn transitions and maternal adaptations, and optimising breastfeeding and maternal–infant attachment, among many processes.

An easy generalisation of this research is that if we leave women alone to birth naturally at the appropriate time, we have a better physiological transition into motherhood. This leans into the fact that our matrescence can be impacted by our birthing process.

I don't share this to shame you or make you feel bad for birthing a certain way. I mean, my first experience of birthing was a physiological nightmare! But if we know this, then we can help ourselves, our child and our attachment to this new babe if everything isn't as straightforward as desired. My first birthing experience was well planned. I did all the 'right' things, and yet I still ended up with a lot of intervention, a lot of drugs and a forceps delivery for my babe. I am sure this contributed to the absence of the love-bomb that I expected to feel — and which I did experience after the natural birth following my second pregnancy.

In the long run, it hasn't impacted my relationship with my child, my connection or my sense of self as a mother, yet because this initially didn't fit into my expectation of how a 'good mother' birthed, I was pretty down on myself (for a good year at least). This needs to be consciously broken down because I feel it is setting mums up for a shame-based beginning to their mothering experience.

One of the great understandings of our shift into matrescence is the role of the mother-baby dyad (a fancy word for duo). In the aforementioned article, Dr Buckley explores beautifully the interrelated physiology that requires both mum and babe to have a beautiful transition. For example, skin-to-skin contact is a hormone-regulation factor; any disturbance to this can affect the physiology of hormones in both the mother and the child.

The combination of this increasing awareness of matrescence as both physiological and psychological is very real and it's becoming a hot topic in the mother-centric circles I mix in. Where is the support for women giving birth who expect it to play out one way only to find it is completely different? We congratulate them on doing it, on the arrival of their baby and on everyone being healthy. There is no decompression from this. There is no discussion about unmet expectations. There is little acknowledgement of the resilience the women have shown in changing direction, most likely rapidly, at a truly vital part of their life.

> *Like waves crashing ashore, our matrescence can be a shore-breaker that leaves no sand particle unturned. It can also be the gentle, soft caress of a small swell onto a quiet beach.*

How it plays out isn't something to be shameful of. The grief we feel as we leave behind our old 'self' is normal.

Bringing an awareness of this matrescence — and the need for conversations among groups of mothers to allow us to grow, magnify and step into our awesome-selves — is a key way that we can embrace the joy and the expansion of ourselves as we traverse this motherhood thing. It is a wonder of motherhood. Encouraging this for ourselves and our communities is vital.

Having the opportunity to reset our motherhood in ways that acknowledge the change — the *who we are* — and knowing how to step forward from it is a key driver of a healthy motherhood. But suppressing the feelings of failure, shame and guilt that can surface during our journey into and during motherhood can impact our health and healing.

‖ PAUSE MOMENT

- Was your birthing experience how you thought it would be?
- What do you wish had been better about it?

Mum-guilt

Mum-guilt is the gift that just keeps on giving. According to discussions with my mum and mother in law, it doesn't necessarily stop when the kids leave home or grow up either. (Sorry to bring that up.) We acknowledge it, we can get rid of it sometimes, yet it just keeps coming back, much like one of those totem tennis balls on a stick. Sometimes it will hit us in the back of the head, sometimes it will surprise us and sneak up from the bottom and other times we can easily bat it away. But unless the string breaks, we can't really get rid of it.

The narrative of motherhood — as I explained in chapter 2 — that says we are suddenly expected to shift away from honouring ourselves and move towards honouring others first is a prime creator of the mum-guilt phenomenon. Cath Sullivan, a researcher of psychological aspects of mindfulness, in her article titled 'Bad mum guilt: the representation of 'work-life balance' in UK women's magazines', explored the role that women's magazines have in decontextualising the guilt associated with the mum-guilt phenomenon, and how they make it a personal, private issue, something mums simply have to put up with because the division of labour is so skewed. What this means in real-speak, is that us saying, 'Hey, I feel bad about not wanting to do all the house stuff and the mum stuff... and I want to go to work instead' should be viewed as a private and personal matter and shouldn't be a matter for discussion.

Reclaiming our 'self' through matrescence is key to allowing us to fully express our life. The role that mum-guilt plays in stopping this can be significant. Mum-guilt is worn as a badge of honour at times. Like, we've all done it, right? It's the ultimate 'perfect mother' myth playing out in our current environment. In a brilliant article in *The Guardian* titled 'Parent trap', writer Eliane Glaser opens with the highly powerful statement, 'Worldwide, mothers are overworked, underpaid, often lonely and made to feel guilty about everything from epidurals to bottle feeding. Fixing this is the unfinished work of feminism'. I couldn't agree more.

The burnout mothers are experiencing in their health and physiology can nearly always be traced back to the experience of attempting to meet the needs of all the peeps around them. Where matrescence in its essence should be about supporting mums to do new things and continue with old ones, it's often in our modern world perceived as an indicator of strength or weakness. It's another tick box of doing things 'the right way'.

There is an understanding that the mum-guilt phenomenon stems from the same components of patriarchal drive that say we are worth the most as a woman when we mother. There is a plethora of toxic positivity around parenting and 'surviving' the early years, and none of it really helps to assuage the mum-guilt.

Let's break it down.

What lies were you told prior to becoming a mum that you can't or won't live up to?

What do you do each day because you should, not because you want to?

What does your soul crave to do?

How does your motherhood journey stack up to your guilt load — is there a disparity?

These are provoking thoughts for mums as they navigate why mum-guilt may be occurring. Bringing an awareness to how we have ended up in the land of mum-guilt and the possible path out of mum-guilt land is a big part of our matrescence.

II PAUSE MOMENT

- Spend some time pondering the questions above. Does mum-guilt show up for you?
- How does it impact you?
- Where is your totem tennis ball at the moment?

The internal shift of a working mum's matrescence

Consciously bringing awareness to the shift that matrescence brings to our big world of working-mum life and allowing us to be all things if we choose to is one of the key reasons I am on this planet. My hope is that by continually bringing hope to the mums of today to demand better support at home, to stand up and speak for themselves and each other and to understand they are not alone, we begin to reclaim our motherhood.

Motherhood can be glorious, healthy, vital and wondrous. We are told that it is hard (sometimes, yes), that there will be struggle (there will) and that there will be boundless love (of course, but it doesn't always feel like this either). Our journey is to recognise that we are a normal, healthy human having a normal, healthy matrescence when we experience all of this and more.

I believe the matrescence of a working mum is different from that of other mums. When we are a personality that has been on the career trajectory, and if we are an older mum, the levels of guilt, martyrdom and possible mental health concerns could possibly be higher.

Being an A type personality who really wants to be the best at everything she possibly can, learning to let go of that to embrace the newness of motherhood is bloody hard work. Because when we are a people pleaser (hello, my hand shoots straight up for that one), we want to do the 'right' thing.

How do we navigate what is the right thing when we have no true north to base it on? Embracing this difficult decision, and honouring that this isn't always easy, is the first and biggest step to looking at how we may need to do things differently from those around us to make this motherhood gig work for us!

Putting yourself first can be the most powerful way to explore matrescence. Let's do this together, beautiful mama!

(4)

THE AMAZING MOTHER BRAIN

Your amazing brain has changed its whole circuitry to allow you to mother in a way that keeps your child alive and improves your connection. It's time we value our phenomenal neurology and self.

One of the little-known facts about chiropractors is that we spend years studying neuroscience, the brain and nerve system function. While we are often identified as biomechanical masters of the spine — which we are — I'd actually be inclined to say that our knowledge of the workings of the incredible master control system of the body is oft underestimated.

The exploration of the amazing mother brain, while not a new topic, is one that is dear to my heart. As someone who inherently understands the beautiful healing capacity of the brain and body, and how we as humans can truly heal from the inside out if we are given an opportunity to do so, I can't help wanting to explain to you how our brain shifts and changes once we become mothers. So even if you think this topic isn't your cup of tea, I urge you to stay with me. Our brain is such an integral part of who we are and understanding how it works will help you get the most out of the 'action' part of the book (parts II and III).

In this chapter, we will explore the different ways our brain works hard to support us in our mothering and motherhood. The main points we will uncover are:

- the magnificent changing mother brain
- vitality, vagus and immune function
- how burnout can show up as brain symptoms (my story)
- helping our brain towards vitality.

Let's enjoy this chapter for what it is...a little bit nerdy. It's a super simplified version of the learnings I've gathered about our marvellous brain over the years, but hopefully it's presented in a way that makes it palatable for you to understand. Enjoy!

The magnificent changing mother brain

I remember when researching the 'mother' brain — our brain during pregnancy right through to the post-partum (after-birth) period — that the common thread was that motherhood changed us inherently for the worse. That having children in fact made us dumber, sillier and unable to concentrate. That it impacted our career choices as we moved through life and that our best was behind us. I knew this couldn't be true because...well, how could it be? Our body is so amazing at knowing exactly what to do when — why would it suddenly drop the ball when we get pregnant and become a childbearing human?

In order to understand this further, I undertook the magnificent 'In Her Brain' course with the most knowledgeable neuroscientist of the female brain I have come across, Dr Sarah McKay. She has a brilliant book that dives deeply into the female brain, *The Women's Brain Book* . This course was an exploration into the female brain, and of course I totally loved the section on how the brain adapts and changes during pregnancy.

Much of the work in this field has been done on rodents as their brains are similar in the way they function to the human brain, providing some super succinct insights. It's a pretty big topic and my goal is to break it down quite simply here for you. If you want specific, intense details, I would highly recommend getting a copy of Dr McKay's book and reading it front to back. Her depth of knowledge is extraordinary.

I am going to detail the key take-homes for the amazing changing mother brain. A knowledge of how awesome it is, how it hasn't abandoned you for better times and how it is constantly working to support you. I found this completely life affirming as I moved to support myself and the mums around me to be the mums that I knew we could be.

The first key take-home I wanted to share is that your brain doesn't abandon you when you get pregnant. The concept of pregnancy brain, or the dumbing down of ourselves once we become pregnant, is definitely a myth I really want to dispel for you.

During pregnancy, our amazing brain refines its circuitry so that it is better able to connect with our unborn child. In the words of McKay, there is shrinkage in 'grey matter in regions of the cortex related to social cognition, empathy and theory of mind'. This allows our brain to work hard to become emotionally ready to read the cues of the unborn child as soon as they enter the world. Our brain basically becomes obsessed with making sure we are able to perform the role of mother.

So our brain does not get dumber — it just changes its focus. I like to explain it as a focus bucket. We can focus on many different things daily prior to mum-life. We can focus on exercise, on what we're eating, on the conversation in front of us, on deciding what we are going to have for dinner tonight. We can easily shift our focus and become aware of what it is we want and need to do to achieve the goals we set ourselves during the course of the day.

If we examine this once we become a mum, our focus, without us even realising why, is inherently linked to our child. Even while I write this chapter, I have thoughts of concern running through my head about my son, who had a small injury at soccer this morning. They just keep popping up — it's my mum brain being intrinsically connected to what is happening in my child's life. My neurology has shifted to allow this explosion in awareness to take place.

If you were working in a busy environment prior to the birth of your child/ren, you probably developed amazing cognitive (learning or learned) abilities that helped you adapt to your work requirements. According to neuroscientist Bradley Voytek, as our brain has approximately 86 billion neurons and is working hard to adapt to our environment constantly, it's probably had a bit of practise at change.

You may have heard the term 'neuroplasticity': the brain's ability to change continually by forming new neural (nerve) connections. Kendra Cherry and Shaheen Lakhan talk about two main types of neuroplasticity: structural and functional. Structural plasticity occurs as a result of learning new things, and functional plasticity is where the brain moves functions from a damaged area to undamaged areas. If you're interested in reading about functional neuroplasticity, I highly recommend two books that explore this topic in detail: *The brain that changes itself* by psychiatrist and psychoanalyst Norman Doidge and *The man who mistook his wife for a hat* by neurologist Oliver Sacks. So perhaps over time, your beautiful brain has altered its functions due to the work that you do and you've become really great at it.

Imagine if we could get our brain to alter its functions like this when we become mums. The research I've outlined above basically tells us that our brain pre-organises itself for success and function during pregnancy and the post-partum period. I mean, if you are someone who likes to get everything sorted before a big event, then you can rest easy that your brain has your back! We are so amazing to be doing this when we become mums. We've just been sold the narrative for so long that we're going to get pregnancy brain and baby brain, and that the altered brain impacts our smarts, that we have likely subconsciously decreased our own worth and value as a result.

Often, as mums, we feel like we exist with a thousand tabs open. Dr Sarah McKay cites Professor Dave Grattan when she says that our brain is adapted to increase its cognition (learning) when we are pregnant and during post-partum periods due to the 'flooding of the brain with the feel-good chemicals oxytocin and prolactin, and 1000-fold higher than usual levels of the cognitive enhancer oestrogen'.

Acknowledging the amazing changes that occur in our brain, and how we are altered neurologically during pregnancy, is the first step. The second is further recognition that this doesn't impact our ability to be ourselves, our smarts or our potential working choices. This monumental change in understanding is a big step forward for females the world over.

❚❚ PAUSE MOMENT

- What is the most revealing aspect of what you've learned about the amazing mama brain?
- How are you grateful for these neurological changes?
- Where can you now sense your brain has adapted perfectly to your motherhood and mothering journey?

Vitality, vagus and our autonomic nervous systems

Neurologically, our body is broken into two distinct systems or parts: the central nervous system and the peripheral nervous system. These are wonderful systems that work cohesively together to support our bodily functions. These systems enable us to move, sleep, digest food and do all of the awesome human things that enable us to live.

We also have a stand-alone system within the peripheral nervous system called the autonomic nervous system. This is the part that regulates our physiological (remember, this means 'bodily') processes, over which we have no control — you'll know these as the ones often called involuntary if you've done a bit of reading on this. This is the part of our nervous system that does all the automatic things that keep us alive day to day. Our breathing, digestion, heart beat and pumping blood, stomach motility... you get the drift. Super important.

When I reflect on the significance of this system and how it pretty much keeps us alive with all of its marvellous functions, I get a bit teary. I think about how it knows, as soon as we are born, to automatically take a big breath. And that if we are born into water, to not do that big breath until we are pulled up and out of the tub. This is the system that turns our food into poo and can somehow decipher corn and not digest it (who hasn't found undigested corn in a kid's nappy?). I mean, it really deserves all the kudos it can get.

The autonomic nervous system

The autonomic nervous system has two components to it: the sympathetic system and the parasympathetic system. I'm going to give you a very simple rundown on these because they're important.

The sympathetic nervous system

This is our fright/flight/freeze system: the one that is responsible for helping us in times of stress and fear.

It's evident when we get overloaded and we get stuck in the 'on' position. The freeze state can be like a form of burnout, where we just don't care about anything and it's easiest to make no decisions. I saw a lot of this after the stress of COVID lockdowns.

Living in sympathetics all the time puts us in a chronically stressed state. This is where we can have physiological changes such as consistently high heart rates, increased oxygen rates, decreased digestion, decreased fertility... the list goes on. There is a brilliant book I recommend to any mum experiencing, or concerned that they are stuck in, this mode. It's called *SD Protocol* and it's by Dr Wayne Todd. He recommends a superb way of resetting your system. There is also a terrific reference book by Dr Libby Weaver called *Rushing women's syndrome* — it's one of my absolute favourites.

These books discuss in detail the impact that rushing and chronic stress can have on our lives. (I'm going to delve into stress in the next chapter.)

The parasympathetic nervous system

The parasympathetic nervous system is responsible for responding to our body's relaxation, resting and feeding state.

These are the great guys we love in our life because they calm us, heal us and allow us to connect to our intuitive state. You might read this and think, yes, I want to stay in this state forever. However, our sympathetics and our parasympathetics are supposed to do a little dance: we are designed to flux between the two. We need both states to keep us healthy. I love my parasympathetic, calm times, but I also love my go time in my sympathetic state. The balance is the juggle that can impact our mama world so much.

The vagus nerve

You need to know the role that the vagus nerve can have in modulating and affecting our amazing mama brain. The vagus nerve regulates our internal organ functions and plays a huge role in controlling our body's response when we are resting and relaxing.

It's our secret weapon for fighting stress and it works by tying together the sympathetics and the parasympathetics in a way that allows us to hack our brain. As mums, being able to easily calm our farm and reclaim that sense of self as things bubble up and over the top is a great skill to have.

I've often seen — in practice and within myself— the vagus nerve serve as a tool that reflects safety and a sense of self back to the brain. The vagus nerve has a beautiful ability to transfer information about our environment back to our brain rapidly. Our brain loves to know that everything is functioning well so that it feels safe. It likes the body to move well to signal safety. The feedback loops from the digestive system, the heart and the lungs through the vagus nerve to the brain are significant in our calm-mama brain state.

Now this may sound like gobbledy-gook, but stay with me. Here's a little story about me and my vagus. At the beginning of 2020 — yes, before COVID — I was accidentally headbutted by my son during a vigorous cuddle. Yep, you know the one: up under the chin where your head jolts backwards quickly. I immediately felt a tingly sensation in my face and thought it would pass. But it didn't.

I quickly got checked, got adjusted, the symptoms diminished and I thought that was it.

Then they came back … along with a very rapid, 10-kilogram weight gain and a lot of facial changes. I thought I had a pituitary gland tumour or a weird form of multiple sclerosis. I did every test under the sun — all clear, thankfully. Yet the symptoms persisted.

Eventually I discovered that, combined with a pesky gut parasite, all my symptoms were related to stress. Yep. Stress. Not the kind of big stress that you think is going to be a problem, the single event that causes you to stop and really understand what stress is. Nope … this was that quiet, slow stress. The type that creeps up on you. The stress that just keeps on keeping on, that lurks in your system underneath all the layers, where you think you have your life together, but you don't really. Not physically or vitally anyway.

I call this the epitome of working mum burnout. That slow burn of stress that emanates from doing all things for all people. Externally, it wasn't impacting my health … until it was.

How did I heal? How did I recover from my burnout? I worked hard on my sympathetic dominance, my gut health and my vagus nerve. In the next chapter I'll be exploring exactly how burnout and stress impact our health. And then in chapters 9 and 10 we'll look at some hacks you can use to regain your health after a significant stress load. I'll be sharing my secrets to achieving this, and hopefully you will be able to heal yourself too. Because you are an innate healing being. You just have to unlock the potential in between all the crazy, busy mama stuff going on!

Back to the vagus. The vagus nerve is a cranial nerve — the 10th cranial nerve, in fact — in our brain stem and it links specifically to the parasympathetic (that's the calm down side) component of the autonomic nervous system. It can impact the control of our mood, immune response, digestion and heart rate. It travels from the top of the neck area all the way down the thorax and into the gut. Research by Breit and colleagues confirms that the 'gut-instinct' feelings we all have relate to the vagus nerve. You see, it's not just made up!

We know from the research (see the reference list for this chapter at the back of the book) that dysfunction in our vagal pathways can be responsible for obesity, anxiety, speech sounds, mood disorders, heart rate, gastrointestinal function and inflammation. How could the vagus be impacting your health? I know when I was at my unhealthiest, the obesity, the anxiety and my heart rate were all affected. My gut problem was due to the parasite, but who knows if this was exacerbated by the dysfunction of my vagus. It's immeasurable, but it always makes me wonder.

As you can imagine, the ability to hack into our parasympathetic function (that's the calm one) through our vagus nerve can be absolutely lifechanging. I've found 10 ways of doing just that. Not all of them are for everyone. You might have a favourite, like me, that helps you reach a calm state quickly. Or you might find several of them work in combination for you. The choice is yours. I'll list them here for you, but we'll explore how they can improve your vitality in chapter 5 because they have a massive impact on your burnout and stress recovery, mama.

My 10 vagus nerve hacks are:

1. cold water immersion

2. singing or chanting

3. yoga

4. meditation

5. positive thoughts and social connection

6. deep, slow breathing

7. laughter

8. probiotics and gut health

9. exercise

10. massage.

Decreasing your overwhelm to enable you to heal is one of the greatest things I can hope to do for you. Your brain and your nervous system are so powerful. By giving you the information to make a shift internally, I can't wait to see your world calm down and explode all at the same time!

II PAUSE MOMENT

- Is there a part of your nervous system function that feels unbalanced?
- How does that show up for you?
- Is your vagus nerve seemingly healthy?
- Which of the 10 vagus hacks jumps off the page for you?

Helping our brain achieve vitality

Parts II and III of this book are dedicated to giving you tools you can use to help your brain function vitally and perform in the best way possible as a mum, and more importantly for yourself. As we've learned in this chapter, our brain really is the functional epicentre, and learning how to unlearn the patriarchal society constraints of mothering, and how to embrace a healthy brain, are two of the best ways we can hack our working mum life.

To keep our brain functioning happily, we know it needs three key things:

- glucose from nutritional foods

- water

- movement.

Glucose and water

These seem pretty simple, don't they? Glucose from food — not lollies (we've all seen toddler brains after too many of those), but the good kind that gets broken down from nutritious food sources. (This is so important that I've devoted a whole chapter in part II to nutrition.)

As US neurosurgeon Dr Imran Fayaz asserts, water is an essential element for positive brain function, with even a 2 per cent decrease in brain hydration causing cognitive delays, and a prolonged dehydration status causing shrinkage of neurons (as we all reach for our water bottles ...). We know that the mental symptoms of dehydration are:

- depression

- afternoon fatigue

- sleep issues

- inability to focus

- lack of mental clarity or brain fog.

I'm sure you've all experienced at least one of these. Did you know that they could be caused by dehydration? There are days, particularly when I'm in the practice with patients all day, where if I don't have my water bottle in the hallway ready to quickly grab in between patients, I don't drink enough. By the time I get home, I'd be lucky to have scratched together 1 litre.

There are also days where I seek out sugar for my end-of-day energy boost, or booze to get me into a perceived calm zone. I wonder how much of this is my brain craving more water, or more neurological input (to make our brain wake up) to keep itself functioning well. I see it all the time among the mums who visit me at my clinic: a lack of hydration, causing them to make bad choices just to give their brain the kick it needs, and to keep them 'up and ready' for the family, is quite endemic.

Movement

We know that movement is vital for the brain to function well. In an article in *Harvard Health*, Dr Srini Pillay explores how moving our body can influence our mental health. This is especially so if we're feeling depressed; in fact, it can be just as effective as medication for some people. A study by brain development researcher Raed Mualem and others identified that movement improves cognitive performance and academic skills, and found that in poorly performing students, it can improve their grades. We also know from literature by one of the world's foremost authorities on the brain–fitness connection, John Ratey, and world-renowned performance psychologist, James Loehr, that movement positively impacts brain function not only around academic performance, but throughout adulthood. Their research highlighted how it improves the 'frontal-lobe mediated cognitive processes, such as planning, scheduling, inhibition and working memory'. I don't know about you, but that sounds like a great relief to me as a mum. Knowing that movement can actually benefit my brain and help other parts of my life that are sometimes difficult to improve is a win–win in my book.

Embracing vitality

Linking the elements of brain health that I've skimmed over here to our inner vitality is where an understanding of how the brain helps us function in our mum-life and working life comes in. Being able to steer clear of ever-present fatigue and overwhelm is vitally important if we want to continue to decrease our tendency to burn out.

Vitality has two definitions, both of which are pertinent to mums in today's society:

- the state of being strong and active, and full of energy

- the capacity for survival, present in all living things.

I love both of these meanings. If I can remain strong and active to be with my kids, my husband and my 'self', then hip f*cking hooray! I've won the life lottery. On a deeper level, if I've managed to somehow unlock the power within me that gives me a sense of life, then that's bloody marvellous too!

As our brain is the master control system for our entire body, understanding how to influence it can change up our vitality internally with intention, which then transfers to changing up our vitality in our external environments.

As we move towards owning our 5 Pillars of Healthy Motherhood (in part II of this book) and understanding the importance of our inner self for good health and wellness, we can bring the concept of vitality and brain function to the forefront. Achieving life-changing health benefits solely by improving our nutrition, increasing our water intake and movement, and subsequently improving our brain function is pretty easy. Let's use this knowledge to change up our mama experience with ease and minimal overwhelm.

‖ PAUSE MOMENT

- How does your brain health stack up when you reflect on symptoms you might be experiencing from lack of one of the three key elements of healthy brain function?

- Which simple tool can you integrate right now to improve your vitality?

- What would being vital look like to you?

(5)

STRESS AND BURNOUT IN MODERN MOTHERHOOD

Modern motherhood is creating generations of stressed, overwhelmed and burned-out mothers, and it's time we reclaimed our motherhood and our 'self' to save our families, communities and world.

Stress is one of the greatest conundrums of modern mum-life. We live in an environment where everyone is busy all the time. Traditional down time has become almost non-existent thanks to phones and watches beeping at us to pay attention constantly (unless we give mindful attention to turning everything off and unplugging).

Our brains were not designed to be in 'go' mode all the time. As we explored in the previous chapter, we need a balance between our sympathetic and parasympathetic nerve systems to maintain health and vitality. Constantly being switched on means our fright/flight/freeze system becomes dominant. With society shifting towards a highly tech- and connectivity-oriented existence, we find ourselves endlessly looking for the next notification, scrolling so we don't miss out on anything and comparing ourselves to the mum down the road, next door or in another country.

In this chapter we are going to explore the effects of stress on mums and how this can lead to burnout. By the end of the chapter I hope you will have a great understanding of:

- the signs of stress in yourself
- calm-state hacks
- how chronic stress is impacting our mothers
- trauma and its impact on us
- motherhood burnout (and how we get there).

Recognising stress and burnout

This chapter doesn't give you the answers to managing stress and burnout (that's coming up just around the corner in part II). What I hope to empower you with here is an understanding of stress and its impacts on your physical body, so that when it comes to changing things up, you'll have an in-depth idea as to why it matters for *you*!

As mums, we cop the constant tech updates from school. The emails. The schedule changes. The family updates. The play dates. The sport and art commitments. And on it goes. Then we throw in tuckshop duty and our own work ... we are always 'on'.

We've forgotten how to stop and just breathe. How to shift our stress mode to the setting we so desperately crave and desire: the 'off' mode. To enable us to shift into our healthiest state, to transform our health and find our connected self we need to:

- stop
- breathe

- be calm

- disconnect

- reconnect

- play

- have fun

- do something we enjoy (like a hobby).

I grew up at a time when *Sex and the City* was a big-deal TV show. If you haven't watched the series, do yourself a favour and check it out because it's all sorts of fab. It follows the lives of four strong female leads navigating their thirties in New York: relationships, marriages (both successful and failed), career, children, sex, cancer.

Here comes a spoiler alert. The main character, Carrie, moves to Paris at the end of the sixth season to be with a man for two reasons: she feels it's the right time to do it, and all her friends have other stuff going on in New York and she's the last one standing. Ironically, she subsequently comes back to New York for the love of her life, Big.

When I reflect upon Carrie moving to another country to chase an ideal that she thinks she needs, abandoning the parts of herself that make her heart sing — Big and NYC — I can't help thinking that her situation is completely transferable to the mother experience of today. We do so many things we think we should be doing because they are the perceived 'right thing' to do. Yet, if we knew how to navigate back to what our soul, our body and our relationships are craving, and what our own heart and being know is right for us, we'd be able to reclaim the lost balance in our lives.

A lot of the stress I see in mums today is focused on the sense of 'loss of self' that we can't quite put our finger on. Combining this with the burnout experience related to our endless to-do lists, our rushing from place to place and feeling we have to tick all the boxes all the time, it's no wonder we have a broken version of motherhood on the rise at the moment.

II PAUSE MOMENT

- When was the last time you embraced the quiet, still, calm space in your world?
- How did it make you feel?
- How often would you like to make it happen?
- What would that mean for you?

How chronic stress is impacting our mothers

Hands up if you weren't impacted in some way by chronic stress during COVID lockdown. It's a well-known fact that chronic stress negatively affects our health and wellbeing. Our body responds to acute stress by releasing stress hormones. A combination of nerve and hormonal signals (and you thought they only affected your period) prompts our adrenal glands to release adrenaline and cortisol (these guys are our stress hormones).

What this means for us is an increased heart rate, elevated blood pressure and a boost in energy supplies from the adrenaline, which gets us moving ready for our stress response. The cortisol increases sugars in the bloodstream, enhances the uptake of glucose via the brain and curbs non-essential fright/flight/freeze reactions. And all of this suppresses the digestive system, reproductive system and growth processes. Not nice.

The amazing thing is that this also communicates with the brain to control mood, motivation and fear. Now I don't know about you, but I'm pretty sure we can say that motherhood (and often pregnancy also) can create a level of chronic stress not previously experienced. Yes or yes? According to PANDA (Perinatal Anxiety & Depression Australia), up to one in seven new mums and one in 10 dads experience postnatal depression in Australia.

We also know that a chronic stress response can put you at greater risk of many health problems, including:

- anxiety

- depression

- digestive problems

- headaches

- heart disease

- sleep problems

- weight gain

- memory and concentration impairment.

What's more, there are known impacts of maternal stress in pregnancy on the foetus. In an article on maternal stress during pregnancy and early childhood development, Matias Berthelon and associates observed that stress possibly affects foetal development. What's more, the importance of a child's first 1000 days from conception is known to impact cognitive (learning) and non-cognitive skills. Children who were exposed to in-utero maternal stress presented at the age of two with a lower level of development, cognition skills and more attention problems than children who had not been exposed to maternal stress. If we can negate this through awareness and skills to navigate our societal expectations of busyness, then we can actively improve the lives of children in generations to come. How awesome is that!

According to the Australian Institute of Family Studies (AIFS), the percentage of parent couples where both partners work has increased steadily, from 53 per cent in 1996 to 61 per cent in 2016. It's estimated that between 2002 and 2015 fathers worked on average 75 hours per week, with 46 hours of paid work, 16 hours of housework and 13 hours of childcare. Mothers worked an average of 77 hours per week, with 20 hours of paid work, 30 hours of household work and 27 hours of childcare. We can see from this data that the 'mother-load' of early years' parenting generally falls squarely on the mothers.

The last time I did a time study to assess where all the time in my week was going, I found I was doing at least — yes, at least — 35 hours per week of housework/child rearing and chauffeuring to and from sport. This was on top of the 30- to 40-hour work weeks I was doing, and the attempt at five to seven hours of exercise. No wonder I was heading towards burnout land.

As mothers who are living this stress-load experience, we need to bring a cognisant awareness. By bringing choices of mindfulness, presence and connection into our day, we can choose something different. Not just doing this with or for our children, but with ourselves, our partner, our tribe and our communities.

Connection is what we truly strive for. Anecdotally, in my practice I often see mothers who feel lonely and isolated in ways that they didn't experience prior to having children. My colleagues and I prioritise the understanding of village, connectivity and social connection as a key pillar of health, and we love to create space for relationships and community to stave off the loneliness epidemic hitting mothers.

When I work with other practitioners to create awareness of supporting mums to overcome the chronic stress elements that cause burnout and ill-health, we primarily address:

- breath work

- movement

- outdoors time

- water and nutrition

- social connection.

For you at home, we are going to dive deeply into the 5 Pillars of Healthy Motherhood, which can support your health to overcome extreme stress and burnout. I know that adding another thing to your plate might feel overwhelming, but through dedicated space creation — and awareness that society is driving you to do things that you feel you 'should' be doing, rather than what needs doing — together we will find some space for you!

‖ PAUSE MOMENT

- How does chronic stress affect your health at the moment?
- How would you like to kick it to the curb?

Motherhood and trauma

I can't write a book during COVID and lockdowns and climate change and misogyny without touching briefly on trauma. I'm not a trauma expert by any means, but I do understand some of the neurology around how it gets embedded into our systems, and how it then traverses our body to affect our soul, our health and our day to day.

If you need support around trauma, I recommend you seek out a professional trauma counsellor, psychologist or psychiatrist who can guide you in working through its impact on your nervous system and your body. One-on-one support to navigate this is vital for healing. My hope is that this section of the chapter opens up some thought processes that will steer you towards the healing path when and if required.

Trauma is defined as either a deeply distressing or disturbing experience or a physical injury. I think, for years, there has been an understanding of the physical elements of trauma: the trauma we can physically see, the specific event that has happened. The responses to these types of events from support people are generally positive because they are tangible events. The knock-ons of that level of support for someone can be huge and neurologically positively lifechanging.

What is difficult to understand within the scope of trauma are the experiences that occur in the day to day, or emotionally, in a person's life: those that can shape their human experience and their view of the world. We see it playing out in large scale in the armed forces — or after someone has suffered a huge life event — in the form of post-traumatic stress disorder.

Yet between these two huge experiences, there is also an undercurrent of trauma happening that creates neurological shift and change over time. According to the US Center for Substance Abuse Treatment, whether a trauma occurs as a result of natural events or by humans impacts the way we react to it. If it is perceived as human-derived trauma, the effect on us is emotionally and behaviourally more traumatic. If it is a large-scale event or a human-caused trauma, we are usually offered assistance in the immediate aftermath. However, our knowledge of the neurological impact over time of smaller scale or prolonged traumas, such as the effects of a pandemic, is limited. We could assume that it began as a natural-based trauma, yet the continued lockdowns, divisiveness and anger in our communities over time could be perceived neurologically as human-caused trauma.

Where this leaves us as mothers working from home, schooling children, managing lives and dealing with all the unknowns of living with a pandemic is anybody's guess. How it relates to burnout, neurological fatigue and ongoing health issues is something we will discover in the next 10 to 20 years.

Trauma is defined as having three distinct categories: natural traumas, accidental/technological catastrophes and intentional acts. It is the intentional acts that cause the greatest stressors around the traumatic experience. In their book *Trauma-Informed Care,* Amanda Evans and Patricia Coccoma list intentional acts as arson, terrorism, sexual assault, homicide, mob violence or rioting, physical abuse or neglect, stabbing, warfare, domestic violence, school violence, and so on. Being a pandemic, COVID and its stressors fit under natural causes; however, some of the acts associated with it in our local communities, where we have seen protesting and mob violence, could fall into the intentional acts category as well. Regardless, bringing an awareness to the overwhelm and stress of our day to day is paramount.

The resilience bucket

Mothers, especially those who have children with special needs or who live in volatile circumstances, constant trauma from living on the edge and walking on eggshells, are undoubtedly affected neurologically over time. Even if you don't define yourself in these terms, have you ever felt like you've had a bad day or week...and then the smallest thing tips you over?

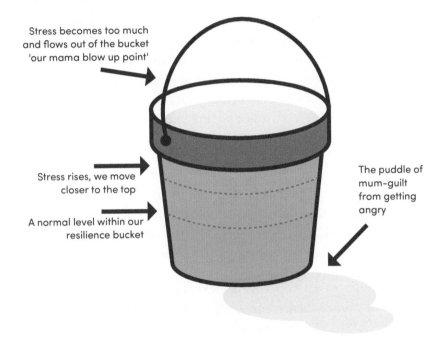

Stress becomes too much and flows out of the bucket 'our mama blow up point'

Stress rises, we move closer to the top

A normal level within our resilience bucket

The puddle of mum-guilt from getting angry

I refer to this as our resilience bucket. It's a combination of trauma and neurological readiness for our day to day. When we are constantly filling it up with small-scale issues, perceived problems and other outside phenomena, and we are unable to unplug the hole in the bottom to let them out, we end up with an overloaded bucket — and that's when we snap. This can come from chronic, low-grade trauma events; it could come from the constancy of the unknown through the pandemic; it could come from the kids always talking and demanding; or it could come from trying to balance your work–life and having to do *everything*.

As mums, we need to learn how to open the hole in our resilience bucket. Bringing awareness to our energy, our values and our needs, and then seeking a tribe of women to create our support network, is how we make awesome brain changes and increase our health, vitality and love for ourselves again.

We know that our brain is super amazing. In his ground-breaking book, *Breaking the habit of being yourself*, renowned author, speaker, researcher and chiropractor Joe Dispenza affirms that the stronger the emotional reaction is to an experience, the higher the emotional intelligence impact (quotient) it creates. What this means in real-speak is that the bigger the 'thing' that happens, and the bigger our reaction to it, the more it creates a cemented or hard-wired pathway in the way our brain responds to this type of 'thing'. This moves forward to create a known circuitry so that the next time you have a big event, your amazing brain remembers its emotional reaction from the previous time, and it does the same thing again.

Basically, it falls back on its known circuitry and creates a response that is comparable. Joe Dispenza says our breakthrough comes in shortening the refractory period that this response holds in our system. By recognising our response, and knowingly shortening the stress in our system, over time, we can alter our stress response to known events or trauma.

This is similar to my concept of knowing when and how to pull the plug out of your resilience bucket. According to the American Institute of Stress (AIS), 33 per cent of people report feeling extreme stress, 77 per cent of people experience stress affecting their physical health and 73 per cent of people have stress that impacts their mental health.

The AIS states that the four main demographics or types of people with the highest rates of stress are:

- ethnic minorities

- women

- single parents

- people responsible for their family's health-care decisions.

With these statistics, we can see how, as mums, we condition our bodies into a state of fear and heightened stress responses. By recognising this, we can see how stress can really impact our resilience, our zest, our calm and our health. Learning and applying the tools to unplug the resilience bucket is something I want you to conquer. And, with my help, you'll be in control of your resilience bucket (all will be revealed in chapter 9).

II PAUSE MOMENT

- What are you biggest stress producers?
- What is your physical response to them?
- What is your emotional response to them?
- What would be your favoured response to them?

Motherhood burnout

Burnout among mums is becoming an increasingly common problem. The chronic stress felt and the huge adaptations made over the COVID lockdown times of 2020 and 2021 influenced our resilience and ability to bounce back from stress for years to come. The World Health Organization (WHO) defines burnout as:

> a syndrome conceptualized as resulting from chronic workplace stress that has not been successfully managed. It is characterized by three dimensions:
>
> - feelings of energy depletion or exhaustion
> - increased mental distance from one's job, or feelings of negativism or cynicism related to one's job
> - reduced professional efficacy.

The WHO adds that this definition refers specifically to stress in an occupational context and not to other areas of life.

I find it highly interesting that the classification specifically relates to occupational stress causing burnout. I guess it's lucky for us mums that mothering is work, and work is work, so we are doubly occupationed up the wazoo!

Let's examine the WHO's three key elements of burnout from a mother's perspective:

- *Feelings of energy depletion and exhaustion.* These are definitely a component of mothering and motherhood. They impact sleep, bring on the chronic 'exhausted' status and make it difficult to garner the energy levels required to keep on functioning. And they can occur at various stages in working mums' lives. This is where we turn to living on caffeine and sugar to support our survival mode.

- *Feeling distanced from our job.* Specifically, we often refer to mentally distancing ourselves from our children or job as an element of post-natal depression (PND). What if it is a significant element of burnout in mothers? What if we are actually getting close to a point of no return, and to overcome the feelings of negativism or cynicism we need support? Because we are undertaking two jobs, we may feel maternal guilt around feeling the burnout emotions. Motherhood really can drive us to doubt ourselves and where we are at relatively quickly if we can't get the support and tools we need.

- *Reduced professional efficacy.* I know there are days when turning up to the office and being professional after not much sleep due to little people is super hard. In the WHO's context, I believe they are insinuating a continual alteration in professional efficacy. If, like me, you are working 30 to 40 hours per week in your job and then being a mother for 30 to 40 hours per week also, the likelihood of decreasing professional function in either of these jobs is high.

The WHO has obviously dedicated resources to this increasing concern of overwork and burnout and its impact on health around the planet. There may be people who read the guidelines and don't believe they fit into this classification because they feel they don't fit into the category of 'working enough'. I'm here to tell you that maybe you work more than you think, and that could most definitely be forming part of the problem.

My top 10 reasons for motherhood burnout

A few years ago, one of my mentors, Brandi MacDonald — a social worker and trauma-informed counsellor who works with chiropractors — wrote an article about how chiropractors were getting burnout in the healing profession. It sparked something within me, and I used this as a basis to write about the 10 ways that we, as mothers, are getting burnout too. I acknowledge Brandi for the kick in the butt to begin me on this writing journey, and the discovery of how we can support ourselves and other people in our orbit.

Here are my top 10 reasons for motherhood burnout.

1. *Boiled frog syndrome.* It creeps up on us like this: we begin by tolerating our own low-level behaviour because it seems minor. We are driven in service to our family; we are driven to have a certain mothering experience and to work a certain way. We have a constant busyness or rush in our day-to-day life, which slowly warms up the pot of water we are sitting in ... which eventually becomes a pot of boiling water that we can't escape from.

2. *Misalignment of our actions.* We behave in ways that don't support how we want to parent — who we want to be as a person — and convince ourselves that it's okay just this one time. We do it for a small period of time, which extends out to the 'normal' things that we do, meaning it continually bleeds our energy — that very special energy that is needed for our health and wellbeing.

3. *Seeking validation.* We are highly charged, emotional beings ... mother beings. Validation is the hardest desire to

fulfill. Do we get it from our children's hugs? Do we get it from ourselves? Do we get it from our spouse/partner? Do we need external validation? Are we constantly doing 'everything' and chasing validation as the end point? Chasing that feeling can create a roundabout of failure and lack of fulfilment.

4. *Not knowing how to care for our mind.* Doing the right things doesn't always equal healing and a thriving life. So we work out, we eat the right things, we get adjusted by the chiropractor, we take all the supplements. Sleep is going to be interrupted because we're parents, but these things should help to sustain us throughout the day. But we're still feeling disconnected from our families, unhappy and unfulfilled. Because the way we view the world, our belief system around what motherhood should look and feel like, the way we view what is happening is distorted. Bringing in the altered belief systems that we have generationally or socially acquired impacts our view or lens of motherhood. We can't out-behave a distorted mind or belief system. We need to address this in our mind, our thinking and our values systems, and look at our core beliefs of motherhood.

5. *Unrealistic expectations about people or events.* We simply don't control what we have been led to believe we do. To me, mum-life provides an opportunity to finally realise this, yet we can easily try to spend our lives seeking to control, chasing that illusion and never succeeding. This is really exhausting, and is part of how we end up creating the desperation and frustrations we may experience in our motherhood. The expectations placed on us by Instagram feeds, by mummy influencers and by other people showing us the good side only — the lack of 'real-ness' in our relationships — creates a 'should' mentality. People are 'shoulding' all over our motherhood experience, and it's unrealistic. It's creating a horror of expectation both within society and internally within ourselves.

6. *Lack of self-care.* Just as in point 4, where we do all the things except look after our mind, in this element of burnout we stop

doing all the things that help us to look after bodies. We stop eating properly, we stop working out, we stop food planning and the sloth behaviour kicks in. Our new reality becomes not looking after ourselves. And then it just continues. This drives the health markers that will increase the stress load and can lead to burnout.

7. *Life is simply entropic.* Entropy is defined as a 'lack of order or predictability; gradual decline into disorder'. In this instance, it also relates to the thermodynamic quality of breakdown as things convert. What this means for us is that if we aren't continually trying to improve ourselves, we will eventually break down. A pretty morbid concept. But as mums, we don't often have the time, or we perceive we don't have the time, to continue to seek constant improvement. Seeking constant improvement doesn't have to be hard work, fatiguing or tiring. But if we don't, we will die a little bit more on the inside because that's what happens — that's the law of life.

8. *Lack of personal responsibility.* When you view the world as something happening *to* you, versus *for* or *because of* you, your life and family become predators and you become a victim. Victims are helpless and hopeless. If this is your truth, it's not long before you feel victimised. We can feel victimised as mums. When we don't get the support that we want, that we feel we need, then we feel we're failing. We feel we're not standing up to the ideals of what we should do because our support networks aren't stepping in. We have the power of knowledge and reflection. Have you actually asked for help? Are you able to acknowledge that maybe all these things are happening to you because things haven't been set up correctly in the first place?

9. *Not having boundaries.* I see a pervasiveness in the mums I work with, the belief that relationships and environments — not they themselves — control their emotions. When emotions control us, our physiology responds accordingly and breaks down to give us more energy, much like the chronic stress and trauma responses discussed earlier. This drives us towards an energy depletion state

because our physiology is responding to an emotional effect, so if we keep depleting that energy in situations and/or with people who continue to bleed us dry energetically (energy vampires), it continues on and on.

10. *Your environment or habits never change.* Sometimes you need to mix it up externally to create an internal mix-up. When we never leave our environment — never change up our routines or habits — we become a frog in water. And this takes us back to point 1 ... and the cascade continues.

I know burnout is real.

You know burnout is real.

We see it every day in our lives. Mums we know and love are burned out in this journey, which should be joyful. They're not giving the time, energy or effort to experience the love side of mothering, they don't know how to ask for support and how to receive it, and society expects so much unpaid and unappreciated work by our mums. We are trying to do everything, instead of just being in the journey and the process.

Sometimes we can't do everything. It's okay to have days where we don't do everything and we curl up into our hibernating selves and reset a little. Survival, and looking after yourself, are really important because you can't look after your family if you don't look after yourself. It's not selfish to look after yourself at all. Not even a little bit. It's a great time now to acknowledge that. It's time to do the work. I can't wait to take you through your journey from burning out to burning bright!

II PAUSE MOMENT

- How has burnout shown up in your life?
- Which of the 10 reasons is one that really resonates with you?
- What can you not wait to change in your world now?

Part II
MAMA

The 5 Pillars of Healthy Motherhood

This is where the fun begins. Woohoo!

So far we've looked at how society is driving your experience of motherhood, why you can choose your own adventure, how your brain can be hacked and how you can get rid of burnout and stress through changing actions and functions — and learning how to love yourself again. It's been a ride. A massive info dump into the parts of motherhood that you may be experiencing in full, partially or not too much at all. My hope is that this has given you a bit of background as we dive into the 'doing' stuff.

In part II we are going to explore the 'how-to' behind helping busy working mums, just like you, who really need support to overcome the burnout and reclaim the zest, joy and health they deserve. Now I know you don't need an extra to-do list item so my goal is to guide you to change out some things for others, rather than making it all bloody hard work.

The basis for all of this is helping you, as a mum, to find simple tools to make you healthy, vibrant, joyful, connected and calm. In my programs,

I teach about my 5 Pillars of Healthy Motherhood: five categories that make the process a bit more streamlined and easy to navigate.

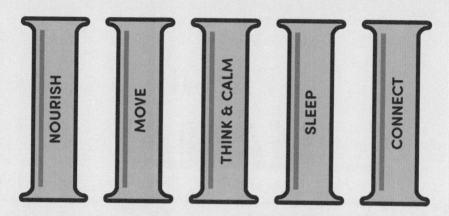

By the end of part II, my hope is that you will have built yourself a toolkit that allows you to choose what is going to work best for you to create the motherhood you desire. If you are looking to gain more out of your motherhood journey than just the usual extra coffee, guilt from mum-fluencers on Instagram and wine-time on a Friday, then you are probably in the right place. Reclamation of your 'self' on this huge mama-journey — and the how-to of achieving that — is the exact reason for this part of this book. I want you to reclaim more for yourself in order to show up as a greater version of who you are and to express your life fully and vitally. That's what the 5 pillars are all about: how you can have more of the things you want.

More can look different for each of us. Maybe more looks like you are healthy and vibrant on the inside, with amazing gut health, quality sleep and energy during the day.

More could look like a reinvigoration of a movement in your system that actually supports you as a mother and doesn't create more ill-health. Maybe it recognises that you have inherently shifted and that your movement patterns should too.

More could look like an appreciation for the importance of social connection and the role this plays in your healthy mother mindset.

That is, the significance this plays in your ability to thrive mentally and emotionally in the mother journey.

More could look like the ability to calm yourself, and possibly the loved ones around you, through your actions, intentions and skillset. More could be your self-talk: your mindset and your ability to turn those days that are full of stinking thinking, and the hormonal interplay this brings, with a mother mind.

More could be sleep. We all want it. But how can we improve it? How can we hack it? How can we discover a version of sleep that operates well for us in mum-zone and serves us now, rather than being a pre-child memory of something we used to have!

More could be that you are able to reclaim your feminine self and honour the woman that you are now in all your beautiful mother glory.

The 5 Pillars of Healthy Motherhood are the simple keys that, as a mum, you can use to simplify your health and vitality journey. These concepts are not new, and I'll fully acknowledge that it's my nearly 20 years in practice working with mums that has allowed me to learn the tips and tricks to make this a workable concept for each of us.

I want to preface this journey with a reminder: you are awesome just as you are. Motherhood hasn't broken you, but society may have driven you to burnout and you may need a way to navigate out of it. I've created a way for you to simply and easily change your world, one pillar at a time, without adding to your to-do lists or your overwhelm, and to be able to simply place yourself at the centre of your world, even if it is just for five minutes a day.

These pillars, when you integrate them, are absolutely life-changing. I can't wait to sink into the details with you!

(6)

TOGETHER WE RISE

The togetherness of mums' souls when they are united as a community or collective is extraordinary.

Togetherness is the glue that keeps us human, creates community and drives our brain to function in a completely different way. (Our brain thrives when other humans do similar things to us at the same time; it thrives on social connection, and it fires more joyful hormones when we're with other people.) Togetherness allows us to explore our own humanity and have a human experience that we may not otherwise get to enjoy. Togetherness is one of the many things that differentiates us from the other species on the planet. As a mum, your 'together people' can form the most life-affirming and supportive relationships you will have. I mean, seriously, who doesn't want to walk into a park and see their gang of wonderful humans smiling back at them (and if you know me, you'll know I'd be late enough that the reality is they would already be there).

We also know that when we have those times where we may not feel together with others, the stark loneliness can be a trigger for mental health problems, feelings of judgement and sadness. Motherhood is a time when being together is one of the most important things on earth.

In this chapter, we are diving into community and collectives. My hope is that it will help you discover the tools and understanding you need to find your community of women, and to embrace them and allow yourself to be embraced by the encouraging women in your world. The top takeaways from this chapter are:

- why belonging to a community is good for your health

- how to discover your values: the *who* behind the *why*

- how to incorporate values into your daily life

- energy stuck-ness and *you* (a how-to of shifting our energy state)

- how to find your village.

As Seth Godin writes in his book *Tribes*, 'a tribe is a group of people connected to one another, connected to a leader, and connected to an idea... A group needs only two things to be a tribe: a shared interest and a way to communicate'. Mums crave this style of community, yet in our busy society it is easily lost or never found to begin with.

In past generations, there was a strong sense of community — of a village 'feel' — that over time has been lost to a large degree. A village of humans who check in on us, who can intuitively tell when we are feeling 'off', who we can lean on as they lean on us when they need support. Even prior to the craziness of COVID, when our world got turned upside down, our society was struggling to keep up with all of the things that were demanded of women. In a 2019 article in the journal *BMJ Open*, Hannah Dahlen and colleagues identified that 30 per cent of Australian women report severe sleep and settling problems with their infants. It is understood that this leads to maternal exhaustion and poor mental and physical health in women, impacting their early mothering experiences.

One of the outcomes of this important work by Dahlen and co. is that mothers need regular mental health assessments in the first 12 months of their mothering journey (with each child). It is vital to have professional check-in moments with our mums as regularly as we do with our children, as well as instilling the importance of togetherness in mothers. Dahlen comments that mothers need to feel more supported. I would like to take it a step further by saying that we really need our 'village' around us in order to feel supported. I know it's become a pandemic buzz-phrase, but the expression 'to lean in' fits so well here. If we have that together feeling around us, we are more likely to feel safe to reach out and ask for help.

Remember when I talked about safety and trauma in part I? How our brain functions in amazing ways when we're feeling safe and nurtured? This is pretty widely accepted at those times when we are knowingly vulnerable, such as when we give birth and in the newborn baby stages, or if we're suffering from post-natal depression (PND). Yet once we are past that newborn phase, we kinda forget about the safety thing.

Imagine the power in having a safety barrier around yourself all the time. How it can transfer to our brain being safe, telling us neurologically that we are safe and that we could function on a whole different safe level.

I feel safest when I know I'm loved, I can sense the love and I have peeps around me. There are many mothers the world over who exist in this space the majority of the time. Woohoo to you if you are one of them. But what about the mamas who don't? That's why check-ins and awareness of support requirements are so vital. That's one of the key reasons why our togetherness matters. Because it signals safety, love and warmth and allows us to grow, be us, be true to ourselves and love in on others as we feel loved in on ourselves.

According to Harvard staff writer Liz Mineo, research conducted over the past 80 years found that while good genes impact longevity, what's more important if you want to feel happy is connection with community. I don't know about you, but I found that when I had young children, having less time available due to my new lifestyle meant I wasn't prioritising community at all. In fact, it was a really hard slog finding a village of women for myself.

During my first pregnancy, as I outlined earlier in the book, we were living overseas with a three week old and there weren't many other expat mums around. The sense of loneliness was real, and I'm sure is part of what thrust me back towards my career and working with other chiropractors virtually. I knew I had a group of practitioners that suited me already out there I could work with. They matched my values, and we had mutual understandings about how we worked and the desire to help kids in our practices. I felt valued, seen and like my old self. In retrospect, I was craving something I really needed.

The togetherness of values

The common sense of value can drive us to establish a community around us. And it's this shift to finding a commonality of values in a world that is currently filled with increasing outrage, loudness and busyness that is proving more difficult. Traditional mothers' groups are wonderful; they allow mums who are all going through the same experience in their mothering at the same time to connect with one another.

The mothers' group experience was lost for most mums during 2020 and much of 2021. The collective coming together to experience the highs and the lows was lost. And this has created a lot of trauma and mental health concerns in the mothers I'm seeing in my practice. While completely different circumstances, this seems similar to my experience of mothering from a distance when we lived in Malaysia. I had phone-in friends in Perth, and my mum and sisters-in-law back in Australia, but the camaraderie of meeting up with other women was sorely lacking. It was pretty bloody lonely.

Community is a huge factor in how much happiness and joy mothers feel. So now we're going to explore what it is we can do to find our peeps again. To find those mums we really want to hang with, bad dance with, sing with, clean up poop with, cry with and laugh with.

Let's go find them!

‖ PAUSE MOMENT

- Where have you felt that you have experienced community and togetherness on your journey? (Is it at mums' group, the doctor's office, with your own family, your friends?)

- Where have you felt it lacking? (Lockdown life? Loneliness? Health concerns?)

- If you had a great village, what would that actually be like for you? (Think about how it may make you feel on the inside, and what would be happening for you to think that way.)

- What would it look like in an ideal mama world in your mind? (Write down all the ways it would be awesome to be a mum in your imaginary perfect world.)

Before you look for a community, find yourself

Now I'm not saying you need to walk around to all the mums on the playground and chat to them like you're in a bar trying to find the love of your life (though I have done that). One of the ways you can go about finding your village initially is to be certain of yourself first. Yep, you are a totally awesome mama and finding yourself is going to be a whole lotta *fun*!

One of the best ways I've found for figuring myself out is to look at my values. What do I stand for and who am I? It may seem a bit daunting, but knowing who we are and what we stand for can be a gamechanger when we are attracting those amazing other mamas into our orbit. There are plenty of resources out there to guide you through all of these things, but let's run through it together here in a way that I've done for years and that ... as yet ... hasn't let me down.

Discovering who we are is something we can do at any stage of life, and it's something that's forever changing. Getting a current snapshot of who you are in your perfect awesome self right now can be really helpful. It can help you dive deeply into what makes you tick.

Determining your values

This exercise is simple in its nature, but can be quite deep in its reality. I remember the first time I did this. I was away at an experiential retreat for work, which basically means you do weird things like build canoes with a team and then sit down and debrief what it meant and how it made you feel.

I loved it.

It opened my eyes to what made me tick on the inside, and more importantly, why that then made me respond in a certain way at certain times. The important work of values changes across your lifespan. This shift in values, in my experience, is never more evident than when you become a mum. With the neurological shift that occurs in our brain, and the way that we are able to step up and into our mothering experience while embracing our matrescence — that beautiful shift of a woman into motherhood — it's no wonder that things change.

So let's get into it!

- *Step 1:* Circle any of the words in the table of values below that resonate with you. Just read each word. Sit with it. Is it for you? Yes! If it isn't ... move on.

- *Step 2:* Group the circled words into similar themes. What are the key ones that stand out for you? Try to create five theme groups — there is no right or wrong with this.

- *Step 3:* Pick your five favourite words — one from each group — that resonates the most with you. These are your values: the top five words for *you*!

Accountability	Awareness	Balance	Beauty
Boldness	Calmness	Cleanliness	Closeness
Commitment	Compassion	Confidence	Connection
Consciousness	Contentment	Cooperation	Courage
Creativity	Decisiveness	Dependability	Determination
Dignity	Diligence	Discipline	Discovery
Diversity	Duty	Education	Effectiveness
Empathy	Encouragement	Excellence	Experience
Expertise	Exploration	Fairness	Faith
Flexibility	Focus	Freedom	Frugality
Fun	Generosity	Gratitude	Growth
Happiness	Health	Honesty	Hopefulness
Humility	Humour	Integrity	Intimacy
Intuition	Kindness	Leadership	Learning
Love	Loyalty	Mindfulness	Moderation
Motivation	Openness	Optimism	Organisation
Originality	Passion	Peacefulness	Persuasiveness
Professionalism	Reason	Resilience	Respect
Sacrifice	Security	Sensitivity	Sensuality
Serenity	Significance	Simplicity	Sincerity
Spirituality	Stability	Strength	Structure
Success	Support	Sympathy	Thoughtfulness
Thrift	Timeliness	Trust	Understanding
Uniqueness	Usefulness	Virtue	Vision
Warmth	Wealth	Wisdom	Worthiness

II PAUSE MOMENT

Once you have your five words—your values—write them down and then answer these three questions:

- How do these values resonate for you? How do they make you feel? Is there an internal feeling of pushback from them at all?

- What, if any, are the surprise words?

- How do you see these in your mama-life right now? Did they fit in your pre-mama life too? What about your working-mama life?

How to incorporate values into your daily life

Now that you know a bit more about what makes you tick (at the present time at least), bring that into the essence of your sense of self on a daily basis. Write these values down somewhere: next to your mirror, in the bathroom, maybe in the car... (I'll tell you how this all fits together in chapter 9.) But trust me, reminding yourself regularly of what matters to you can be a game changer in the long run.

There is a beautiful quote by Ralph Waldo Emerson that defines success perfectly and that I think parlays into this whole value of motherhood thing:

To laugh often and much; to win the respect of intelligent people and the affection of children; to earn the appreciation of honest critics and endure the betrayal of false friends; to appreciate beauty; to find the best in others; to leave the world a bit better, whether by a healthy child, a garden patch, or a redeemed social condition; to know even one life has breathed easier because you have lived. This is to have succeeded.

Your values don't define you, but they do give you an idea of what truly matters to you. Here are mine:

- family

- joy

- health

- connection

- success.

My number one value is family. I love to do things and live life joyfully with my family. Health really matters to me (I know, not surprising), as does human connection. But success threw me. Yes, I know I'm driven, but it makes me understand more about why I love the balance of my work and life. Why I'm a happier mum when I'm able to have success through service to others. Why 'working mum' and 'business owner' are really important for my sense of self, my brain and my joy in the world. Being in service, and successful, when I am filling my own cup to help fill that of others: this is where I feel amazing. If I exist only as 'a mum', I am a very unhappy human.

Sometimes, my success value jumps right up to the top, and we have a little value-off in our house because my husband would totally love it if my number 1 was family all the way, every day! But there are days and weeks and seasons where that isn't right for me. Learning this about myself — that it didn't make me a bad mum, that it was just an essence of my human expression — allowed me to be more at peace with who I am and how I can support others while being true to myself.

How about you?

It's not selfish to honour what is your true self inside.

Finding those things out — the things that make you tick — going out there and doing them … that's when you will begin to attract your community. When you are happy and connected to your own good self...that's when you will be happy and connected to people in your orbit too. A study conducted by Rebekka Kesberg and Johannes Keller linked our values to our experience of life, and while it wasn't conclusive, it found that our values help us interpret our surroundings and the situations we find ourselves in. But what does this actually mean for us as mums?

Maybe some crazy thing happens at the park with the kids. Maybe one of them thinks they are funny and splashes water or ice cream or popcorn all over another. Now if your values are joy and fun, you might laugh (though some might find that inappropriate). If your value is cleanliness and order, you may find it tougher to see the funny side. If your value is a strong sense of discipline, you may work hard with the kids to see why it's a problem. If your value is attachment parenting, you may sit with them, have a discussion and try to see the situation from various angles.

There's no right or wrong; it's just different viewpoints. And maybe, just maybe, you'll meet a mum who has the same response as you...because your values match. How beautiful is that? Here's a list of places where I've made friends because of my values (I wonder if any of these work for you too):

- *playground:* laughing inappropriately at my kid falling off something at the park (no injury, just funny)

- *health food store:* organic food

- *skate park:* as a skater mum watching the kids

- *mums' group:* over lunchboxes and WTF to put in them

- *mums' group:* over kids' clothes (coz they are cute)

- *bootcamp for mums:* over exercise

- *conferences:* at the back of the room, breastfeeding

- *coffee shop:* coz coffee is life

- *school pick-up and drop-off:* always late running into the other late mums, knowing looks and eventually we catch up and chat at a school function somewhere

- *playground:* at the top of a climbing frame when the kids can't get down (#activefamilies)

- *online business world:* all striving for more success.

Our values impact all the ways we do things in life. The way they are expressed is impacted by the other four pillars of healthy motherhood, which we will get to in the next four chapters. In the overwhelm of mum-land, understanding our values can be a life-changing moment that allows us to just take a back step and a big breath. It can help us to realise why we are responding in certain ways, why we do things a particular way and why we seem to be in the same stuck behaviour pattern.

When our outside world doesn't match our inside world we can end up with an energy block, and anger and frustration are more likely to bubble up into our space. When we are actioning things that are not congruent with our inner self it can cause friction. I would love nothing more than for more mums to be able to find that inner friction point, release it and find ways to live congruently in their experience.

‖ PAUSE MOMENT

- How can you see values influencing your experience of life?

- Where is your friction point in your values?

- How will recognising your values in the day to day bring the magic?

- Where may values decrease stress and overwhelm for you now?

Energy, stuck-ness and *you*

Who feels they have amazing jump-out-of-bed energy days, and then the ones where you are dragging yourself around one step at a time? Me too! We all have them. Imagine if we could figure out how to shift this when and if we needed too... without it having to be an hour-long meditation, a 45-minute cardio session or a green smoothie that we just don't want. Ha ha.

One of the most difficult elements of this mothering game is that we can get stuck in our bottom-of-the-barrel energy quandary. You know, the one where there is this stuck feeling of dankness within us. Sometimes we can't shift our negative thoughts and behaviours. There are many people the world over who have worked with the concept of our energy driving our human experience, and how if we can turn it around, we can make a change in our day.

In fact, the concept of energy as a large part of our human life form has existed for ever. If we look at the Eastern philosophies that drive the chakra concept, they have been around since between 1500 and 500 BCE according to an Indian text book called *The Vedas*. Chakras are the elements of the body that need to be in balance energetically for us to be in balance in our human existence.

You'll recall me praising the work of Joe Dispenza in the previous chapter. He has a modern take on energy, and for me it is one of the most influential interpretations in understanding how our body can be both whole within itself and generous in the present moment. He writes about the awareness of being who we are and where our energy state is at, and why. Setting ourselves up for the day and being consciously aware of where our state — the state of mindfulness — is at is a way we can shift this energy.

How does this link to our values? As I mentioned above, we can develop an internal friction point if our values aren't matching our actions, and this creates energy drains and stuck points, more commonly referred to as stress and overwhelm. So let's move along with this overwhelm, shake the energy tree and get ourselves aligned again.

The hormones of stress down-regulate genes and affect our immune response.

Our thoughts can make us sick.

Can our thoughts make us well?

How you think and how you feel is how you create your state of being, according to Joe Dispenza. He states that once we hit 35 years of age, we have a hardwired set of habits, behaviours and functions that create our day (breaking the habit of being yourself). So if we want to change our habits, we need to mindfully and with awareness choose different things for ourselves.

This means that as mums and as humans we can choose to make a change, to move our energy, to stop our stinking thinking... but we have to come at it mindfully. I help you do a lot of the work for this in chapter 9. But here's a little pause point for you.

One per cent of our day is 14.5 minutes. That's not very long. If we want to make a mindful shift in our behaviour, or do something that supports our energy, then we can do this through choosing 1 per cent of our day to be different. Bringing a meditation practice in. Journaling. Sitting outside or inside quietly. Doing the thing that shifts our energy state. Dancing. Singing. Running on the spot. It doesn't have to be quiet; it has to be chosen. For you.

As we mindfully think about where our values sit in our everyday, and where we can choose our 14.5 minutes to purposefully craft out our existence, even in the busy mum-world, we sense the possibilities and feel our body change. Where are you feeling the tension? Where are you feeling the ease?

When I reflect on my values — and my body and my life and my busy — I realise that when I'm snappy with the kids or my husband it's because I'm living out of congruence. It's when my energy isn't getting its flow on. It's when I haven't looked after my health and I'm tired, or craving sugar and caffeine. It's when I haven't had any fun and play in my world for a while.

It's when I feel I'm all mum, and I have no business owner time. And it's when I haven't had time to fill my own cup.

All of these reasons for energy stuck-ness are valid and real. The sooner we can step up and honour ourselves as mums, the greater our experience can be...and hopefully the less crank and overwhelm we'll see in our day to day.

II PAUSE MOMENT

- Where do you feel your energy gets stuck? (For me, it's in my shoulders physically and I notice it most when I feel 'stuck' in the kitchen.)

- How would you like your energy to feel? (Vibrant, bright, burning, bubbling, contained, explosive?)

- What would this mean for you? How would an energy shift change your world?

Finding your village

So, we've discovered your values, we've unstuck your energy. Now, how the hell do we find our people? I'm going to get a little woowoo on you again here, but have you ever heard the expression, 'Your vibe attracts your tribe'?

This is never more noticeable than in mum-land. Once we know what we stand for ourselves, we will pretty quickly work out which peeps we meet who do and don't fit our soul. I always recommend that a great place to start is at your local mothers' group. If you have a newborn baby, then getting involved in your local mums' group is a great way to meet a local support group. I craved this as a new mum, and very luckily slotted into one when we moved back to Australia.

Many mums meet through social meet-ups via Facebook or Instagram. Or they know that attachment parenting is something they value highly, so they go to the local babywearing group. Maybe you highly value organic food. I know mums who have found great friends through the local health and organic shop. Finding our support circle based on who we *are* — not who we *think* we *should* be — is an awesome place to start.

Your collective of awesome humans will begin to show up when you are open to it and you are confident in yourself: playgroups, mothers' groups, church groups, exercise groups, bootcamps, your chiropractor's office (yep, it has totally happened in our front room) . . .

I promise you, the village will show up when you are confident in who you are. It's also really important for me to say here that you will probably lose some friends along the way. You can't be there for everyone, and the choices you have made and the stage of life you are in can really impact your older friendships too.

I have been very blessed that a lot of my older friendships have stood the test of time and blossomed into beautiful mama support networks that I can rely on. I mean, these are the girls who were there when I got dumped unceremoniously, when I left all my underwear drying on a heater in Berlin, when I flew back to Australia at the age of 21, when I met my husband . . . yep, those kinda girls.

But I also collected a new community along the way. I started with my exercise girls: the other mums in the mums' group who wanted to go walking or do a HIIT class in the front yard while the kids played on mats. I collected beautiful mamas who were passionate about the food they feed themselves and their children, and the holistic philosophy they bring to that, but who also like a champers on occasion too — coz, balance, right?

I've collected a tribe of professional mums who, like me, were displaced into expat life when their partners were moved internationally for work. We all bonded because we had to try to do the same things like figure out a new country, schools, food, exercise and community in a foreign land.

At no stage did I search; they turned up at times when I was ready and open for it. But it was always when I was focused on something. My exercise crew turned up when I really wanted to regain my fitness. My food crew when I was challenged with what to eat. And my expat crew was a whole new experience.

Some of my village live close by; many of them don't. It sucks, but I guess that is part of the human experience. I know that when we come together, when we exist in this human experience and we find our people, our brain lights up differently. We respond differently. And this is the power of community.

I would love for you to understand deeply to your core where you are at, and then to begin to express that in your day to day. You will find your people. Your village will rise. You will do this together. Motherhood is an expression of village that we have forgotten. My hope is that you can regain the collective of women around you to support you, and for you to support them. To feel that joy when you walk into a room and you know that your people get you! That enveloped sense of calm and of a solid soul.

(7)

NOURISHMENT

As a mother, nourishing our souls with food can be one of the great joys that helps us bring together our family and our community, and inspires our sense of self.

There is so much conflicting advice on food, nourishment and the 'shoulds' around healthy eating. I think, initially, we need to strip it back to what its essence is. The purpose of food should be to nourish us. To keep our system whole and our body working towards homeostasis (the balance of all the chemicals and functions in our body). Food provides the nutrients we need for our cells to keep functioning and it flushes out toxins. Happy eating is the awesome joy that comes from tasting something super perfectly delicious — and preferably not from your kids' leftovers.

There are many resource books with extensive advice about maternal nutrition, and I've popped a few of my favourites in the reference section. I am not a nutritionist, and I make no claims to be. But I do know that the key for mums is to keep things simple. You might find that seeking specific, personalised advice from a qualified nutritionist, dietitian or naturopath is the best option for you.

In this chapter, I will present a simple, wholefoods-based approach to nutrition for mums. I'll explore:

- why food matters
- the power of wholefoods
- what macros are (carbs, proteins and fats)
- integrating wholefoods without increasing stress load.

Plus, I've included a cheeky recipe collection for you in the appendix of the book!

Our matrescence body's metabolism and how we may need to nourish ourselves is different from what we might be accustomed to. For periods of time, our food not only supports us, but also our children through placental exchange and breastfeeding. Not to speak of the energy required of mothers, and how we need to nourish ourselves so we can show up as our best.

The trick is to know how to approach this because there is so much shame around food. Shame is defined by renowned author Brené Brown as an 'intensely painful feeling or experience of believing that we are flawed and therefore unworthy of love and belonging'. It's an emotion that affects all of us and can profoundly shape the way we interact in the world.

Shame around food can play out in many different ways. It can play out as us feeling unworthy of healthy food because why should we care when we already feel or look a certain way. It could play out as a flaw because we keep choosing unhealthy food rather than sticking to our guns and choosing well once we've decided to do so.

Shame could even show up because we don't know how to effectively nourish ourselves, and we feel bad that we need to seek out support in this area. It's not shameful, it's just recognising that we don't have all the answers ... and we most definitely do *not*.

There are so many mums out there who have invested a bunch of time and energy into this, and that's super awesome.

There's also a bunch of mums out there who have no idea or no time to invest in figuring out all the hard stuff. I mean, seriously. Which book do we buy? Which influencer do we listen to? As a mum, is it low carb, no carb, high fat, no fat, no sugar, natural sugars? The questions are endless, right?

Our discussion around food is going to focus on a few key factors, and these are the ones I want you to have a think about as we progress towards integrating some simple key changes into your life to reset and reclaim your motherhood.

- *Wholefoods are key.* Our body is designed to absorb from sources that are as close to their natural state as possible. So if it grew, or walked, or quacked, or flew or swam ... that's the kinda stuff that is going to nourish us.

- *As mums, particularly, we need all the macros.* That is, we need protein, fats and carbs. Yes, everybody is different. However, these things are vital for survival. And removing whole macro groups from your diet is likely to mess with your system (sorry to the low-carb and no-carb mamas. If it works for you, keep going with it).

- *Having a balanced view of food is vital.* We need to foster a relationship with food that supports ease and nourishment. There is no point if it all seems too hard to cook, to source, to nourish, and so on.

- *Food can be fun.* Let's bring that back into our family dynamic.

And that's it. We are going to focus on these elements to really bring us back to learning to love our food, and through this, love our bodies and nourish our souls. Imagine how much more energy we could have to show up in our day to day if we nourished our body with a state of ease where it wasn't hard to do. Where it was supportive, functional, easy for the family and achievable.

‖ PAUSE MOMENT

- What do you currently think about food? Is it a part of your day that brings you joy and ease, or is it really tricky and does it fill you with dread? Is it an annoying factor for you?

- What would you like to do differently regarding your food choices?

- How would this improve your relationship with food, and what would be your expected outcome from this?

Why food matters to me

Let's start with some of my complicated food journeys. I honestly believe that my years of learning, trialling and rabbit-hole jumping led to periods in my life where I had a dysfunctional relationship with food. None more so than when I was mothering.

To lay down a bit of the backstory, I grew up on a farm where my mum and dad cooked food that came from animals on our land, local families or supermarkets — the old-school type that often came from local producers. In retrospect, it was a pretty idyllic way to learn about food.

From these simple beginnings, combined with my love of travel, my love of cooking and food began. Yet despite all this, in my mid-twenties in particular, I began having reactions to lots of my favourite foods, and it was determined I was most likely coeliac (or at least strongly gluten intolerant). In the following couple of years, 12 other coeliacs were identified in my family, which led to the beginning of a different way of eating. I began restricting a lot of stuff, and focusing on healing my dysfunctional gut through diet.

Which is a great thing to do. However, it's so easy to take it too far. And I'm pretty confident I did.

I would go through cycles where I would shed weight by taking all of the food out of my world, and then slowly slip back into a similar cycle of eating again. I would stay off gluten, but ebb and flow between no carbs, lots of nuts and seeds, high fat, low fat, paleo, keto, dairy free, full dairy, juice fasting... you get the picture.

And it served me well for small periods of time, but it wasn't sustainable. It definitely led to me having binge moments that created a real cycle for me around bingeing, restricting and repeating. Interestingly, I'm not the only mum in my world who has experienced this. We've all been on the diet train, right? My hope is that we can create sustainable nourishment in the mum-world that is easy, simple and supportive of the hormone systems of post-partum mothers as they progress through life. A little caveat here: this is really general advice based on my personal experience and in practice with my patients. This isn't advice for you specifically, and if you feel you need to get more information in this area, seek out a nutrition support provider who works with post-partum mothers and understands their needs.

In the past, I built up my picture of healthy eating through assessments including blood tests, stool analyses and DNA testing. Finding a practitioner who can assess you in this way if you feel you need that next level of support is a great thing. And, interestingly, as I researched this topic extensively, a lot of the information is about what the pregnant mother should eat in order to create healthy offspring, yet the post-partum research is still lacking in lots of ways.

The power of wholefoods

Stepping into the power of general wholefood-eating philosophies, the keys to our nourishment are:

- ease
- simplicity
- low stress
- affordability.

Let's take a good look at this.

It is so easy for us to reach for the quick fix of packaged food, the sweet treat or the caffeine load in order to get us through the day. And it's these poor-quality, nutrient-poor foods that can really impact our health in the long term.

Creating ease and simplicity for mums around how and what we eat is key. Changing our narrative from not eating well enough to how we can support our mums to choose differently is key. My intention here is not to create more work for mums, but to streamline their food consumption and preparation so that choosing healthy works for the whole family.

As I mentioned earlier, we need a full spectrum of protein, carbs and fats. According to my beautiful friend and female nutrition expert Sarah Hopkins, most mums are scared of carbs and are not eating enough protein. It's pretty hard to get the protein in at different times, so we're going to examine these three key areas, and how we can support ourselves to choose healthy food easily.

Carbohydrates

Carbohydrates are not your enemy. In fact, eating wholefood-quality carbs is essential for living. According to the Australian Dietary Guidelines, we should be eating from the five food groups:

- vegetables
- fruit
- grains and cereals
- meat (preferably lean)
- dairy.

How we distribute this food intake is really important for us as mums though. We know if we are breastfeeding, that we burn on average an extra 500 cal/day, which needs to be considered in our dietary intake. We also know that we need nutrient-dense foods in these categories, rather than the poor-quality processed foods that we can find in each of them.

According to dietitian Lee Crosby:

> Carbohydrates are an important part of a healthy diet. But some people consider all carbs, from soda to sweet potatoes, to be equal. Decades of science tell us that this simply isn't true—the body handles lentils differently than it does lollipops.

(*Sugars—especially the refined type—are definitely problematic in the carbohydrate-loading world.*)

So how do we get carbohydrates from real food sources? We get them from vegetables, grains and fruits. We get them from real food that contains carbohydrates. I know for me, as a highly gluten intolerant mama, it's often easier to get them from a packaged 'gluten-free' product, yet all of the extras added in with the carbohydrate load aren't great (more to come on that later).

Carbohydrate sources for busy mums include:

- oats
- potatoes — sweet/white/red
- quinoa
- pulses (beans, lentils, chickpeas etc.)
- pumpkin, parsnips etc.
- buckwheat
- beetroot
- bananas

- carrots/vegetables

- taro and cassava (if these are local to you; be mindful of transport. Ease of finding is key. In all my years of living overseas and in Oz, I've never found them outside areas where they were indigenous)

- rice (preferably brown)

- spelt flour

- wheat flour.

A few things to note here. There is a lot of colour. This isn't by mistake. The colours are vital for our health. I know when I'm busy, I reach for the same few carbs... potato and pumpkin, with some beetroot thrown in sometimes. I'm scarred from years of low carb and try to avoid grains — but, if we use wholegrains that aren't super processed they nourish us well. The red veggies are important because they each bring different minerals, vitamins and antioxidants into our gut system. These red veggies aren't always on our radar, but adding them in when we can is really great for their prebiotic properties, their seeding for a healthy gut and their antioxidants.

Where do big, green, leafy vegetables fit into this mix? Much like the red vegetables, they bring us goodness. They are rich in vitamins A, C, E and K, and some of them totally rock the B vitamins (mustard greens, broccoli and bok choy in particular). The dark greens also provide a significant amount of folate, which is great for our cardiovascular health and in preventing certain birth defects. These super veggies also help in decreasing our cancer risk and increase our fibre intake without overloading our carbohydrate content.

As for the heavier carbohydrate-loading foods — the rices and grains — it's great to incorporate these into our diets, as they seriously nourish our soul and our gut system. Keeping away from the white varieties provides great balance and keeps it less processed... which has to be a good thing, right? Because don't our bodies love things in their natural state where possible?

Using a variety of carbohydrate sources and combining proteins with carbs is the key to healthy nourishment, as my beautiful powerhouse friend Sarah Hopkins says. I keep the heavier, denser carbs for a few times a week, and fully load myself on all of those yummy vegetable-based carbs the rest of the week. Nourishment from the inside out helps me to be connected and soulful with what my body needs.

I used to be scared of carbohydrates, thinking they were the devil for my health, but mindful awareness and creating ease in my week for food preparation allows them to be nourishing in more ways than one!

II PAUSE MOMENT

- What carbohydrate source can you take out of your diet that is highly processed and harder to digest?

- What carbohydrate source can you *easily* add in that will support a nourished gut system?

Proteins

These guys are what we, as mums, can often struggle to get enough of. The thought of prepping our protein load can be really tricky, and time consuming, and let's face it, the kids don't always love protein either.

So what are proteins? Basically, they are the building blocks of our cells. We need proteins to build our new cells, to help our kids develop, to aid in the growth of our placenta and the foetus and to support us as we nourish ourselves and our children, whether or not we breastfeed.

Proteins come in many different shapes and sizes, but there are some really simple ones. Eggs are great, but not everybody tolerates a lot of eggs. I know I used to eat bucketloads of eggs, but when I decided to give my body a rest from them for a while, I realised how much they were contributing to my bloat and inflammation markers, like puffy eyes (yep, seriously, it was so crazy) — particularly if I ate them every day.

So just like the three main food groups, variety is really key. Too much of any one thing can't be great for us, and just as with carbs, we want to find a way to enjoy our proteins in as natural a way as possible.

I get protein in my day by eating:

- eggs
- collagen sprinkled on other foods, like oats or in my morning cuppa
- chicken
- turkey
- beef
- lamb
- kangaroo
- venison
- veal
- fish
- nuts
- tofu (this one can be a bit controversial due to it being based on soy curds, but like everything, moderation is still the key)
- milk/yoghurt/cheese
- legumes/beans.

According to the Better Health Channel, women need 2.5 serves of protein per day. So what is a serve of protein? They define one serve as:

- 65 g cooked lean meats such as beef, lamb, veal, pork, goat or kangaroo (about 90 g to 100 g raw)

- 80 g cooked lean poultry such as chicken or turkey (100 g raw)

- 100 g cooked fish fillet (about 115 g raw weight) or one small can of fish

- 2 large eggs

- 1 cup (150 g) cooked dried beans, lentils, chickpeas, split peas or canned beans (preferably with no added salt)

- 170 g tofu

- 30 g nuts, seeds, peanut or almond butter, tahini or other nut or seed paste (no added salt).

So, in busy-mum land, what can this look like? We could have some eggs or oats with collagen for breakfast. We might have a chicken salad for lunch with some pre-cooked roasted veggies (with the colours of the rainbow), some green, leafy vegetables and a bit of dressing. Then we might have an afternoon snack of fruit and a few pieces of cheese. And then, for dinner, we might have a cook-up of veggies and a small steak, a lamb chop or some fish.

The great thing about wholefoods is that if we spend a few minutes on the weekend planning our week, we can easily get our protein, carbohydrates and fats in ... it's just a matter of making it work for us. In my busy world, I tend to have two 'prep' days in the week. This isn't about having to prep for a whole day — it's just getting some stuff sorted so when I'm busy, I don't have to think. I'll run you through this at the end of the chapter, after we've had our chat about fats.

II PAUSE MOMENT

- Where are you needing more protein in your day? Which meal screams 'protein needed'?

- Which protein source do you think will be easy for you to add into your day?

Fats

I remember growing up in the 80s when everything went low fat. Because fat was seen as a killer of people…or something along those lines. I remember seeing low-fat ads on the TV, and I had a thigh-trimmer exercise thingy and skipping ropes. Total 80s kid right here. The research at that time was all about how fat clogged our arteries, caused cholesterol imbalance, and contributed to heart attacks and strokes. And yes, we know that too many of the not-great fats are what can really impact our weight load. Those trans-fats — you know the ones they use to cook chips and to bulk up our processed foods — are quite inflammatory.

Before we go any further, let's have a little bit of a chat about inflammation. In a 2015 article, nutritionist and exercise physiologist Kevin Fritsche explores the concept of inflammation playing a central role in the chronic diseases we are seeing in our modern world. The increase in dietary fats impacts our immune system and alters our inflammatory status. He explores how saturated fatty acids, in large quantities, really amp up the inflammatory quota, and while, like me, you may get outward signs of this such as puffy eyes or bloaty feelings, it's really the inflammation on the inside that we need to worry about. When we are busy mamas, we can easily turn to easy-to-buy processed foods, but unfortunately they are more likely to have the types of fats that drive up inflammation.

One of the reasons that vegetable oils are perceived to increase inflammation is their high levels of omega 6. We know that we need both omega 3 and omega 6 in our systems as essential fatty acids, and we have to consume these through food because our body can't produce them naturally. In nature, these omegas are often present in a 1:1 type ratio; however, over the past century, this has increased to as much as 20:1, as stated in a 2016 article by Artemis Simopoulos in the US journal *Nutrients*. Joseph R Hibbeln and associates support the burgeoning research indicating this shift towards high levels of omega 6s contributing to the chronic inflammation we are seeing in Western society.

Chronic inflammation in our beautiful mama-community may present as:

- obesity

- heart disease

- cancer

- Type 2 diabetes

- arthritis

- irritable bowel syndrome (IBS).

We also know that poly-unsaturated fats are prone to oxidation. These fats have increased bonds in their cell structure, so when they are used to create the cells in your body, it increases their susceptibility to oxidation, meaning that you have more free radicals coursing through your system and oxidative stress occurring. Basically, these are nasty pac-men travelling around your system, rather than the nice guys. We don't want them ... and they are no good for us.

So what does all this mean?

It means that we have choices around the fats we consume. We need them for survival, but some are better than others. In a nutshell, the following list shows the ones to avoid due to their higher level of omega 6s, both in your pantry, and in processed foods:

- soybean oil

- corn oil

- cottonseed oil

- sunflower oil

- peanut oil

- sesame oil

- rice bran oil.

If we can replace them with better sources of fats and have a balance where possible in our omegas, then we can really change the nourishment value in our diet and decrease inflammation, aches, bloating and those god-damn stoggy feelings.

So the good fats: what do they look like for us?

According to Michael Joseph, founder of the website Nutrition Advance, the use of wholefood fats rather than oils is ideal for our body to uptake well. There is a bit of debate in the nutrition world about the digestibility of the fats in some nuts, so trying to find other ways to get the fats, and not relying wholly on nuts and seeds, is important.

This list, which is by no means exhaustive, gives you an idea of different foods that include balanced and digestible fats for our mum-system:

- avocado
- egg
- fatty fish (tuna, mackerel, salmon, sardines)
- chia seeds
- flaxseeds (and flaxseed oil, not heated — my go-to on salads)
- nuts (macadamias, walnuts, almonds)
- olives
- olive oil
- tofu
- yoghurt and cheese
- coconut and coconut oil.

Incorporating these fats into our diet regularly can help our brains, our cells, our inflammation rates and our digestive system.

II PAUSE MOMENT

- Are there some sneaky high-omega-6 fats in your diet that you can easily stop eating to decrease your inflammation load?

- Which two of the healthy fats can you add into your week?

Let's now look at how we can incorporate healthy food choices into our diet.

Integrating food choices into reality

So as a mum, this is seriously the hardest part. There's probably not a whole heap I've just run through that you don't already understand and that you haven't been exposed to before. It's not new research that has just come up ... it's just a whole lotta common sense packaged into a few pages in a book for mums.

But where the magic comes in is making it work for mums in the day to day. We all have brilliant intentions around eating well, and supporting our own health and that of our family through food choices, but it can be bloody hard work when life happens.

As I mentioned, I do a lot of prep work to make it achievable for my family to eat wholefoods in a conscious way. I spend a few hours on a Sunday and again on a Wednesday just getting it all ready. When I cook a main meal, and particularly if I'm roasting veggies like sweet potatoes, I'll always do an extra tray of roasted veggies ready to pop into salads.

I don't love leftovers for lunch, but I do love the ability to make life simple on my busy mornings.

Here's a sample prep session:

- On Sundays I make a batch of healthy biscuits for the lunchboxes — often an oat/cinnamon/apple/dark choc chip type of scenario. I use gluten-free or spelt flour. This gives the kids something to munch on that's not out of a packet. I cook a meal on Sunday nights (I love a Sunday roast) that provides leftover protein for salads the next day. I soak some oats to increase their digestibility (particularly for me), ready to turn into porridge the next morning for brekky. I include lots of veggies in my food shop and I often make two days' worth of salads for my husband and me for work so that I know we aren't reaching for the stuff that's easier to grab in the mornings.

- Trying to be mindful of protein in the mornings and the importance of mastication (chewing, not that other fun stuff), I make up some ham and egg cups on Sundays so they are ready to go for brekky on the run the next day, or I pre-make a protein smoothie. When I do this, I use a combination of protein powder and collagen. (Ideally, I wouldn't use a protein powder for this; however, sometimes it is just easier to do it that way.)

- On weekday mornings I make porridge with collagen, honey and some fresh fruit or eggs with a bit of avocado for brekky. If I'm having eggs, I'll try to add a heathy piece of spelt bread or some roast veggies on the side to get that balance of carbs and proteins into the start of the day.

- Because I eat my brekky around 7 am, I have a mid-morning snack between patients — generally a smoothie (with collagen powder to up the protein content) and the salad I prepped the night before for lunch.

- Afternoon tea in the car with the kids is fruit, maybe a few nuts or peanut butter, or a few pieces of cheese.

- Then we have dinner, which is often pretty boring. Meat and veggies (I'm very lucky to have meat and veggie eaters in my house). We vary it up depending on the day. For example, on Tuesdays my husband drives the kids home because I'm still in practice. So, we try to keep this a simple night in the kitchen. I pre-cut veggies for baking or steaming and have a quick-cook meat available. Sometimes I marinate some chicken or have some sizzle steak ready to go.

- I do utilise my slow cooker/instant pot a lot. I find the convenience of getting home from school/sport at 4.30 or 5.00 pm to a delicious, cooked pot of chicken drumsticks or beef curry can't be overlooked.

Some other great ways that I get a balance of protein, carbs and fat are:

- *soups*. We love chicken and vegetable soup, pumpkin soup (and I sometimes shred some protein into it or have it as a starter), with a protein afterwards.

- *stir fries*. These are quick and easy. My kids are slowly growing to love them and it is super simple to get a great balance of nutrition into them. Having them with some brown rice and enough protein, combined with the veggies, is great.

- *home-made chicken nuggets*. If you have picky eaters, these can be a godsend. Chicken mince, minced veggies, some cheese, roll them in buckwheat flour and bake in the oven. Delicious, and gets all the good stuff in.

- *spaghetti bolognese*. I recently heard about shaving small pieces of liver into the sauce. A massive gamechanger for me, and it ups the nutrient value of this Australian staple.

- *baked ham and egg cups*. I began making these in South Korea as an easy brekky meal and still come back to them as a grab and go.

- *broth and poached eggs with greens*. This was a yummy weekend brekky we often made when we lived overseas. Using a homemade chicken broth, and popping it on the stove with a couple of poached eggs in it and some fresh leafy greens, ups the nutrient value and is quite warming on those winter days.

- *simple salads*. You can add so much colour to your salads. Different cabbages, lettuces, capsicums. You can use some basic healthy oils, some herbs and different proteins.

It can be simple; it's a matter of finding what works for you.

In the appendix you will find some recipes to get you started. These recipes aren't balanced by a nutritionist and if you are aiming for super balance in your world, I'd highly recommend getting a personalised nutrition plan. However, they work in busy-mum world, and for that reason I can't wait for you to give them a go!

(8)

MOVE LIKE
A MOTHER

Move like you love that God-damn body that your mama gave you.

Movement is one of the best ways to change a mama's world. As far as the 5 Pillars of Healthy Motherhood go, well, this one goes close to being my favourite. And I think the reason is, the results I feel in my body are massive, and they happen immediately.

I'm not saying that I suddenly get a six-pack (I've never had one of those — kudos to anyone who has). I'm talking about that inner feeling of shift in energy and sense of self when we have moved our body. We know that our brain, as well as our body, thrives on movement, which offers so many amazing ways to reset our day.

One of the best and most under-utilised tools we can use to look after our brain is to move our body. One of the key ways we can unplug our resilience bucket and let some of the stagnant energy, thoughts and feelings that are just waiting to spill over out through the bottom is through movement. I don't know about you, but that's a 'hell yeah' from me.

In this chapter, we will explore the ways that, as mums, we can support our health through movement. You will gain an understanding of:

- pelvic floors, birth trauma and how it can happen
- fatigue, energy and when to move
- the five ways movement is important when we are mums
- adrenal function, HIIT workouts and rest
- safe exercises for pelvic floor function.

When we enter our season of motherhood, which in my opinion never ends, we inherently shift our body forever. This matrescence — shifting of a woman to a mother — is a never-ending change. And with it comes some physical changes. Regardless of how we give birth, our pelvis undergoes changes that can characteristically alter it moving forward. Our method of birthing does impact the integrity of it for some women, while others can bounce back with little changes.

Let me give you my example as we navigate movement. Prior to having kids, I was pretty darn fit. I played a lot of touch football, found running 10 kilometres a few times a week fun and really enjoyed the gym and Pilates. I was working in a busy practice and I found movement necessary to keep my body ticking along in a way to support my practice.

Once I became pregnant, I felt intuitively that I needed to stop running at about 12 weeks and switched to a brisk walk and then a waddle. That was just me. I have friends who have gone right up to 36 weeks and maintained their running and crazy cross-fit protocols. I kept up with Pilates and gym until we moved to Malaysia when I was 20 weeks pregnant.

We lived in a compound and were not encouraged to walk outside of it, so I cut laps in there early in the mornings to avoid the heat, went to the gym and swam in the pool. It was great. When I was ready to give birth for the first time, I felt physically prepared. I'd done a fair bit of hypnobirthing work due to a fly-away comment from a radiologist when

I was 15 who said that I wouldn't be able to have a baby naturally because of my scoliosis (well, I showed him). At 35+6 weeks, I flew home to Perth ready to nest and prepare for our babe. Having worked with pregnant women, mothers and kids for years in my practice, I really wanted my baby to have a natural birth. In fact, I placed way too much pressure on myself to do this, which I'm sure impacted my birthing outcome.

My daughter decided to come a little later than expected at 41+1 weeks (eight days past the due date). The whole process was long. I had a hind leak of waters, managed at home and then went into the family birthing centre. Eventually, with no signs of go-time (after quite a number of days), I ended up having a chemical induction, 12 hours of labour, lots of unwanted examinations (this is a topic for another day) and an epidural. I was wheeled to theatre expecting to have a caesarean and ended up with a third-degree episiotomy and forceps delivery.

I'm sure I'm not alone in this. In fact, I know I'm not.

What this did to my pelvic floor health, and my ability to exercise the way I did prior to my pregnancy and delivery, was quite significant. We moved back to Malaysia two to three weeks after this traumatic experience so I didn't get a six-week check-up with the physician who performed the episiotomy. I had no physiotherapy to help support my recovery. I relied solely on feeling 'okay' to guide my return to exercise.

After my daughter was born, everything seemed okay. I was back in the gym doing light weights about eight weeks post-partum, and back running at about four months. There were no significant issues. I had a review with a women's health physiotherapist when I got back to Australia. I had to do some exercises to support my recovery further and she altered a few of the gym moves.

Then I got pregnant again.

During this pregnancy, I worked through until 37 weeks, adjusting people, leaning consistently in one direction and probably not resting enough as I was trying to do everything. We moved house when I was about 38 weeks pregnant, and I went into spontaneous labour at

41 weeks. This labour was textbook amazing. I call George's birth my healing birth. It was completely unassisted, transitioned well and he went straight from my womb onto my chest. A slight graze and no other trauma to the pelvic floor.

Hooray!

I thought I was home and hosed. Because I didn't have any specific injury during that birth, I decided I could get back into things like I did the first time. I didn't take into consideration the considerable stress of having two kids under two. My husband was out of the house for work for 14 hours a day. My family lived 3000 kilometres away, but I did have my husband's family nearby for support. And a community ... I had a great community who supported me.

I started back under the guidance of a PT, as I had a diastasis recti — abdominal separation — that I wanted to work on healing. I also started running, most likely against my intuitive gut instinct, but I thought, *if I could do it last time, I sure as hell can do it this time.* I did it with a double pram and two giant kids. Altogether, they would have weighed close to 40 kilograms. And we lived on a big hill. I didn't start back running until four months post-partum — but I still remember the day I really felt my pelvic floor give way.

One day, I ran along flat ground. I ran down a hill and across a bumpy park with both kids in the double pram. I turned left to head along the river path on a relatively straight section. I was about 600 metres from home, and I'd definitely emptied my bladder before I left. I then got the urge to go again ... never a good sign. So I slowed down to walk for a while. I began running again, and instead of the urge, I had a full incontinence leak. I couldn't hold it. It was like my pelvic floor had lost all the ability to hold anything in.

I was really wet. To my knees.

This gave me a few realisations. One, I knew I needed some more specialised help for my pelvic floor. And two, I obviously wasn't voiding or emptying effectively. Both of these can be problems after you have kids. I mean seriously, who remembers that first wee after you give birth to your babe? Holy moly.

I sought help, got exercises, tried all the complementary things to heal it. It would go through phases, and I got back to running with some support at certain times of my cycle, once my breastfeeding journey had stopped. Yet, it still wasn't right.

I eventually had to seek the guidance of a urogynecologist to have a surgical repair done. It's pretty good now. I'm mindful of it and I can run up to 10 kilometres without it fatiguing out. But I know that it's changed, and this difference is part of my personal motherhood journey. I used to be really angry and frustrated at how this had played out for me, but now I have realised, this is my season.

This season is different for me. And maybe how you chose to move before you were a mother is different from now. Maybe that's physical. Maybe that's emotional. Maybe that's fatigue.

All of those reasons are valid.

II PAUSE MOMENT

- What season of life are you in right now with your physical movement?
- Do you have an element of your matrescence or birthing recovery that may have changed your movement?
- What movement do you love to do in the past and now?

Fatigue, energy and movement

One of the greatest challenges of motherhood for many mums is that the desire to exercise might be there, but we are too tired or time poor to get it happening. Now I'm a massive proponent of the philosophy that movement changes our brain function, but sometimes it's bloody hard to get our bodies moving, get that first movement session in and get the endorphin hit happening to make us want to give it another go.

When we're getting woken up a few times a night to feed the baby, our fatigue load is high. And then, if your kids are like mine, our day starts at around 5 am.

If this is a pattern that's familiar to you, then heading out for a 10-kilometre run or a massive bootcamp session could be a bit problematic. Research identifies a risk of injury if you exercise when you are fatigued. In an article by Sheila Dugan and Walter Frontera fatigue is classified as brain and muscular fatigue, and in the realms of the tired mother, brain fatigue definitely hits the spot. The article states that muscle injury, and in particular muscle strain, is linked to fatigue.

Being mindful of our fatigue is vital.

However, we also know that movement is really important to wake up our brain. To shift our energy, to get a bit of zing back in our day! As a new mum, when I was getting woken up six times per night, I always found if I could move my body during the day I would feel a million bucks compared to the days I didn't get to it. There's a great article by mind-body connection psychologist Kelly McGonigal in Berkeley's *Greater Good Magazine* called 'Five surprising ways exercise changes your brain'. I'm going to share the concepts here because they are all sorts of amazing!

(1) Exercise for connection

We all know what a mood booster exercise is. Not only does exercise produce endorphins, it also stimulates the 'don't worry, be happy' brain chemicals (the same ones mimicked by pot), which helps to reduce anxiety and provide contentment. The best part is that exercise has been shown to prime us to connect with others by increasing the pleasure we derive from being around other people.

(2) Exercise to make your brain happier

The reward centres of the brain (the ones that allow us to feel pleasure and motivation and maintain hope) are given a bit of a jolt when we exercise. If we can include regular exercise in our routines, we actually get more dopamine, and we also create more receptors for it ... so it's like we've been able to make more joy points in our brain! Win! And when we are in that stressed out and overwhelmed mum mode, anything we can do to dial down the sympathetics is awesome!

(3) Exercise to make you braver

If we can create a new exercise habit (this doesn't mean a new exercise, just the habit for it), it enhances the reward system in our brain and also increases neural connectivity in the part of the brain that calms anxiety. Regular exercise can alter the default state of our nervous system so that it becomes less prone to fight, flight or fright.

(4) Move with others to build trust and belonging

My favourite quote in McGonigal's article is from French sociologist Émile Durkheim who wrote in 1912, 'collective effervescence describes the euphoric self-transcendence individuals feel when they move together in ritual prayer or work'. This is why dance classes, yoga or group exercise classes are so great. For mums, this is wonderful because the endorphins released help us with bonding too. I know for me, even a family walk can promote conversation, dial back the crazy and allow deeper connection.

(5) Exercise to transform your self-image

The brain's ability to sense where we are in space (proprioception) not only allows us to stay safe, but it is also important for our self-concept; that is, 'how you think about who you are and how you imagine others see you'. Participating in any physical activity gives us a sense of 'self' in the moment.

***

These five concepts and brain improvements can be implemented by you, mama. It doesn't have to be big movement, just anything that gets your body going. Even if you are fatigued, a short walk around the block, a YouTube dancing video, something that supports your system to have some of these brain changes could be the beginning of something regular that makes all the difference to your brain and body!

II PAUSE MOMENT

- Which of these five reasons for improved brain function from exercise excite you?

- Imagine waking up on your most fatigued morning. What one thing can you imagine doing to move your body? Write it down. Stick it on the fridge. Let's see you start to choose to change!

Adrenals, rest and HIIT workouts

Not to go against the grain too much, but heavy-arsed HIIT workouts may not be serving you well. There is a lot of chitter chatter in the world about our adrenals, stress and burnout. Yet, when it comes to exercise, there are definitely styles of exercise that can really impact us if we are in this category of burnout (or just simple chronic overwhelm/stress).

In a review of overtraining, exercise and adrenal insufficiency, authors Brooks and Carter observe that chronic stress from overtraining can result in adrenal insufficiency. We also know that the literature links stress to ill health and that the essential brain adaptations in the perinatal period of motherhood are influenced by stress events. All of this tells us what we innately already know: motherhood can be stressful.

Fatigue and stress are two reasons why I think we need to be more mindful of our motherhood space. If we are adrenally insufficient, or not bouncing back and chronically stressed (and as I said earlier, make sure you see a great medical practitioner to sort through this), then doing a HIIT workout, or other high intensity training, could just blow you out. I mean, if your bucket isn't coping with day-to-day life, then adding in a physically stressful workout may mean that your bucket completely overflows from the combo of exercise and life. It may not. Maybe that workout pulls your plug, but being mindful that it may be too much at certain seasons in your motherhood is important.

Let me share a story with you. I was chatting to Emily (not her real name), a busy mum, one day, and she was discussing how she had been really stressed. Coffee wasn't hitting the mark; in fact, it was making her more tired. She wasn't sleeping well, and she felt that the overwhelm was very real in her world. With three boys keeping her busy, she was trying hard to do everything and it was burning her out. She was waking up every night between 2 am and 4 am for no reason (a sure sign of the cortisol hormone doing funky things). She decided she might get back into exercise.

She went down to the local cross-fit gym. She knew a lot of the other mums there who were thriving, it was a relatively short amount of time out of her day and she felt comfortable in the environment. She started with some intro classes, got her form looking pretty good and then started attending the main classes. She initially felt a heap of muscle fatigue, which she obviously expected as she hadn't exercised like that in a long time.

But it worsened. Over the following weeks, she started getting severe headaches and significant muscle concerns after each workout. Eventually, she decided to stop, as it was clearly not working for her. She went to her GP and through some hormone and blood testing, they determined she had an adrenal insufficiency. The type of exercise she was doing was exacerbating the problem.

Her medical practitioner recommended slow, steady and purposeful movements for longer time periods for a lower heart rate during exercise.

And this got me thinking. How often, as mums, do we engage in bootcamp- and HIIT-style workouts that we think are going to give us our bodies back, a phenomenon that I personally am very charged about. We think we are doing the right thing by pushing ourselves over short time periods when maybe we aren't ready for that yet.

It doesn't mean the time won't come, but when we are in the state of chronic stress that motherhood can sometimes bring, maybe a slower jog, yoga, Pilates, dance class, barre class, even a not-too-heavy and personally checked weights programs might be best.

II PAUSE MOMENT

- Have you ever felt the level of adrenal fatigue that Emily in the story had?

- Is your current exercise serving you, or creating more stress in your system?

Safe exercise and pelvic floor function

It's amazing how in our day and age, and even with an educated background like mine, we can, as women, still damage our pelvic floors after giving birth to the point of requiring surgery. There are many health professionals out there who do a great job of working with women to check, and then heal, strengthen and coordinate pelvic floor function. In particular though, the first stop is a women's health physiotherapist or physical therapist. These amazing practitioners have the skillset to check for coordination of muscles, lifting and relaxing effectiveness and the role that these play in stabilising our pelvis.

Our pelvic floor muscles are the sling and support mechanisms for our entire pelvic organ load. Understandably, as we become pregnant and our uterus increases in weight and size, they are placed under a considerable amount of stress. I'm not saying that we shouldn't exercise during pregnancy and afterwards — in fact, I know it's vital for our ongoing continence and health — but doing it with mindfulness for our health and pelvic floor status is essential.

The known indicators of a weakened pelvic floor as outlined by the Australian Physiotherapy Association in March 2021 are:

- symptoms of heaviness, dragging, bulge or pressure, which can indicate a pelvic organ prolapse

- urinary incontinence: an involuntary loss of urine. Women are more impacted than men, although it can happen to both genders. It is related to child birth, but also to menopause, obesity and certain types of neurological and musculoskeletal conditions and can occur post-surgically

- bowel control issues causing faecal or anal incontinence, which affects 2 to 20 per cent of the general population. Risk factors for this are obstetric birth injuries (third or fourth degree tears), chronic constipation, a history of bowel surgery and some IBS-style concerns

- persistent pelvic pain anywhere between the umbilicus and the mid-thigh. This can interfere with pelvic muscle function and is commonly associated with depression and anxiety.

Having an after-birth check with a trained physio who can provide targeted muscle training can help avoid urine leakage after having a baby.

In 2019, Szumilewicz and colleagues reported on research of the pelvic floor conducted on 97 women. They identified that undertaking a prescriptive exercise program with a combination of low- and high-intensity exercise combined with pelvic floor muscle exercises if you were already able to functionally use your pelvic floor well during pregnancy improved your pelvic floor function.

Safe exercise recommendations after pregnancy and giving birth used to look something like this: if it feels okay at six weeks post-partum, then you are good to go. If something doesn't feel right, then stop that and try something else. If you used to do the exercise prior to your pregnancy, then you should be okay to do it afterwards as well.

Nowadays, safe exercise recommendations are quite different. I prefer to look at safe exercise recommendations as truly needing to seek out some professional guidance prior to returning to exercise, particularly if you have had a tough delivery, medical instruments were used during delivery or you had a caesarean. Ensuring you know if you have great pelvic floor integrity, and if your abdominal wall has a separation, can really direct your exercise patterning.

Regardless, generally starting with low force and minimal impact is the way to go. In the early days, being mindful of hills or a heavy pram will help you decrease the likelihood of overloading your pelvic floor as you return to your exercise journey. Sometimes a gentle weights program is a great place to start, but getting guidance on that is essential too. I personally loved returning to Pilates with a qualified instructor who modified it for my abdominal separation. It made my life so much easier when getting that core strength back.

I think bringing awareness to your pelvic floor is important to ensure that you are setting yourself up for a future with movement. Your brain needs it. Your kids need it. And most importantly, you need it.

II PAUSE MOMENT

- How has birthing impacted your pelvic floor?
- Do you have any of the symptoms listed above that may need further investigation?
- What support and/or exercise can you integrate to aid your pelvic health?

Moving like a mother

Hopefully you have realised that movement is essential for healthy function of your whole self, not just physically, but mentally and emotionally. It can drive connection, it can set you up for a great day, and it can connect you to your collective of other mums and peeps: to those glorious people you love who have your back.

I know movement is a key part of my mothering. It helps me gain a sense of self when I'm really feeling hard pushed and down in the world. Mum-movement doesn't have to look a certain way. It can be easy. It can be 10 minutes in my loungeroom in my pyjamas. Or it can be a walk or run with the kids and dog.

To be honest, it's often in my pyjamas in the early mornings, or a sneaky little walk or run in the spare 30 minutes I have before I get the kids from school. It's rarely pretty; it certainly doesn't have coordinated outfits to go with it, but it is often combined with a soundtrack from my youth to give me that sparky buzz of memories.

I know that when I consciously allocate time for it in my day, it is about 80 per cent more likely to happen than if I just assume I will make time somewhere. It's kind of like journaling and choosing to eat well. There has to be a bit of a plan at play to allow me to get the movement kick that I need in my system.

I've put together some ideal movements for mums at www.workmamalife. com. Make sure you go and check them out as I update them regularly. I don't want this to be hard for you. I want this to be so very easy it becomes an unconscious inclusion in your day. I want it to be a choice that you know makes a difference in your life.

You are worth the time investment mama-bear. It's not about making yourself look different or weight loss or muscle gain. It's about your soul. Your soul craves movement. And when we honour that, big things can happen.

(9)

THINK LIKE A CALM MUM

Shifting our crazy to calm, our anxious to deep breaths, and our reactiveness to connection—this is where the power lies in our motherhood!

The power in our thoughts and our ability to tap into calm is one of the great ways we can reclaim our health and our 'self' as mums. It can be tricky some days, and a pain in the %#* on others. You get the drift.

The overwhelm and stress we are often faced with in everyday life can create a litany of positive responses or a spiral of stinking thinking. Bringing awareness to our own self-talk and how we can change our thoughts and embrace calm is a massive shift. In this chapter, we are going to have a look at how you can change your inner world to change your outer world.

For some, this topic may bring up concerns, and I implore you to seek professional advice if needed. Sharing this chapter with a friend can also make it seem less hard. And if it's easy for you, maybe you could chat about it with one of your mama friends who may be having a tough time.

By the end of the chapter, you should have a much greater understanding of the how-to of thinking like a calm mum, especially:

- self-talk and the field of positive psychology
- a three-step process to put positive self-talk into action
- mindset and motherhood: chasing the calm
- the seven ways to bring calm in daily
- the power of calm in a crazy world
- affirmations for a calm motherhood
- breathing in 'calm' in motherhood.

We've all had tough times. Those of us who have succeeded in putting together a toolkit of ways to think like a calm mum have probably dealt with some shit in their time. I mean, really in it. I've had days where I thought, *WTAF is going on here?* I've leaned hard into my wise friends, as they have leaned on me. I have undertaken personal development, self-talk work, journaling and made a heap of mistakes on the way.

All of it has worked to help me get to a place where I flip my lid less. I feel more connected with the kids, and I can recognise when I need an outside space for myself or a deep breath and reset. My hope for you is that, on your path to choosing a vital, healthy and joyful motherhood away from the crazy of lockdowns and burnout, you end up with tools you can draw on at those times of stress, overwhelm, meltdown and struggle. Tools that will help you celebrate yourself, show up when you want to and embrace your glorious self!

Self-talk

Self-talk is those conversations we have with ourselves in our head. Those little things we hear when we look in the mirror, make a winning business deal, cake, nappy change or anything we are proud of, really. It's also that little voice that can niggle in our ear when we look in the mirror and tell us we aren't enough, or we should be this or that. Our ability to tap into this and to explore the way we converse with ourselves can help turn a crappy day into something a bit better.

Imagine that you had someone following you around all day telling you that you are fat, to put that food down, to try harder, that what you're doing isn't good enough, the kids don't love you, if you do this you will mean more to them, you should be happy, enjoy yourself...

How would it make you feel? Pretty shitty! Imagine if somebody followed one of your kids around saying mean things to them all day. I'm pretty sure your mama tiger would come out. And absolutely rightly so.

Now, imagine that you have a cheerleader following you around all day saying things like *You've got this! Keep on going! You are doing a great job. You are an amazing mum! Great choice! Kick arse! You look beautiful today! Great effort on going for that walk! Your arse looks great in those pants!*

Just reading that makes me happy; it makes my spirit soar and makes me think I should jump in front of the mirror and tell myself these things right now! It makes me think that all I want for my kids is a friendship group that does this for them. A teacher who is positive in their environment to guide and support them. If we want this for the people we love most in our world, why don't we crave it for ourselves?

What if I told you that you have the power to be your own cheerleader.

And it can be life changing. Woot woot! Bring it!

Positive psychology

The field of positive psychology is ever evolving. In a nutshell, it is about looking at psychology and how our mind works in a positive framework, and how this positivity can impact other areas of our life. The Mayo Clinic has a brilliant paper about how we can reduce stress just by changing our self-talk (I'll detail this a bit further down). I mean, wowser! That sounds amazing! We can embrace positive thinking by choosing to look at the positives instead of the negatives in any situation: it's a pretty simple equation. Taking this positivity into the constant stream of conversation that is going on in our head can really change the way we get our thoughts in order and alter the way we view the world.

Having the ability to switch into positive mode and out of the self-critical mode that is so easy for mums to fall into is a learnt skill. I have worked with mums through the years who have been able to up-level and change their life just through this simple reset. Here are the three basic steps, to follow, according to Brené Brown, when trying to relearn our self-critical thinking.

Step 1: Recognise your negative thoughts

Placing a lens over our thought patterns to identify if they are negative or positive is the first step. I found myself negatively saying *f*ck my life* under my breath whenever something happened that I didn't love. This was creating a really negative jolt in my system, and, interestingly, from here I would feel my cortisol or stress hormones spike and everything just seemed harder.

You may catch yourself doing one of these things:

- *Personalising:* Automatically blaming yourself when something bad occurs. Someone cancels a play date at the park: it's because they don't want to be with you.

- *Polarising:* Things are either good or bad — you are either the perfect mum or the terrible mum, and there is little space for the good enough mother paradigm in the middle.

- *Filtering:* While achieving great things throughout a day, you instead filter those out and focus on what didn't happen or how you could do better or more tomorrow. In mum-land, if you feed the kids, move your body and get some work done, you are winning at life.

- *Catastrophising:* Anticipating the worst even when there is no disaster. In practice, I call this looking for zebras in a field of horses. How are you doing this in your day to day? The childcare centre rings you and immediately your brain shifts to assume that your child has been taken to hospital with anaphylaxis or a broken arm, when it's much more likely that they have a sniffle, they need a new change of clothes or your payment hasn't gone through.

II PAUSE MOMENT

- Write down the negative thoughts that have crept into your brain in the past few weeks and months.

- As you write them, really listen to your body and how it makes you feel as you repeat them out loud.

- Is this a feeling you enjoy having?

Step 2: Challenge the negative thoughts

You are now beginning to identify when these negative thoughts pop into your zone. The ones telling you that you are not doing a good enough job, the world is ending and nobody likes you. The next step is to challenge these. How can you choose to change your thought pattern as it happens?

Identifying and stopping the thought as it happens, when repeated time and time again, will become second nature. The thought will likely still pop up every now and then, but you have a choice to accept it once you recognise it or change it. Let me show you some examples.

I'm a loser: I couldn't get the whole house cleaned today.	**can become**	I did so well getting the bathroom done today. I'm proud I found the time.
What a failure as a mum: the kids are having chicken nuggets for dinner again.	**can become**	My kids are eating food and they are alive.
F*ck my life.	**can become**	Love my life!
I'm always late. I'm late again. Why can't I get it together?	**can become**	I am full of purpose. I will do better tomorrow with being on time. It's okay to be late this time.

II PAUSE MOMENT

- Write down some of your negative thought patterns and alternatives you could use to challenge them.
- Which of these will be the easiest to embrace?
- Which *one* do you commit to include in your day *today*?

Step 3: Put the positive into practice

Using your new-found positive self-talk sentences, let's start putting them into practice. This is creating a new habit in your day, and it won't happen overnight. As I mentioned, the Mayo Clinic has a beautiful framework that I want to share with you:

- *Identify areas to change:* Using the pause moment above, identify where you want to engage in more positive thinking.

- *Check in with yourself:* Periodically throughout the day (I've used alarms to do this), check in with your mindset. Where are you at? It may help to journal this with your pause moments.

- *Laugh about it:* Bringing a laughing and joyful humour to what could be tough at first can really change the practice. And who doesn't feel positive after they've had a good belly laugh? Learning to laugh at ourselves or difficult situations can be a gamechanger.

- *Surround yourself with positive people:* If you have the opportunity to do so, cultivating a positive environment around you can make this conscious shift easier.

- *Tell yourself you are awesome every damn day*: But seriously ... practise positive self-talk every day. What can you be positive about today? Your voice is the most constant one you will hear throughout your life; empower yourself with the choice of what you want to say to yourself.

‖ PAUSE MOMENT

- Which of these positive thinking elements will be easy for you to implement?
- Write down five things you would love to say to yourself every day.

Mindset and motherhood: chasing calm

Mindset during motherhood is a massive component of thinking like a calm mum. The craving for calm in our day can be a very real thing and the mindset around our calm is a factor we can't ignore. Calm can be impacted by our cycle, our kids, the moon, what side of the bed we woke up on ... many different factors. The calmest mums I know still have days where they aren't calm, but the thing I do notice is they have a mindful recognition of this and do things to change it up a bit.

I used to hate nothing more than being told to 'be calm' or to 'calm down'. I wasn't always the most calm child, and being busy and '*up*' is one of my life's gifts. I clearly remember as a child sitting in church on many a Sunday morning with Mum's or Dad's hand on my leg telling me quietly to calm down. I was always excited by what was happening. I was a bit of a know-it-all, so I always wanted to share my answers with whoever would listen. I wanted to do my best and be my best, and I was very excited about all of these prospects.

It also means that as I've got older, due to my nature, I've had to learn to cultivate calm in my world: chasing some quiet space for connection, most importantly with myself so that I'm better able to show up for the people who matter in my world. This is one of my greatest learnings.

By now, we are pretty aware what the burnout state is, where we are told that physically we can't keep going on the way we have been. The relentless pursuit of our values and our dreams, of our mothering pursuits or our turning up to show up for everyone but ourselves has eventually meant that we can't keep going.

In chapter 4 I shared the story about me, my headbutting son, my vagus and stress. What started with an innocuous head bump from my son aggravated what's called occipital neuralgia. It felt like I had ants crawling across my scalp at the back of my head. This settled down after some chiropractic care, and about a week later, I noticed a tingling sensation on my face and my whole face would turn bright red at times. I also gained 10 kilograms in three months — a definite sign of imbalance.

I was so scared that I might have a pituitary gland tumour. Or MS. Sometimes knowing what symptoms actually mean can be more scary than not, take it from me. I was also going through a highly stressful period at home, and business was booming in my practice, so it was all systems go. Things had continued to build up over time, and now my body was telling me what I needed to hear.

After many tests, we discovered I had a gut parasite that was seemingly causing some weird inflammation and the facial changes. Over the course of a few months of cleanses and nutritionist support, I was able to lose the 10 kilograms, heal my gut and stop the facial sensations.

But this wasn't enough. I realised that something else had to give. And that something was my calm point. I had forgotten how to embrace calm in my day. In my week. In my month. I had been pushing on in service and forgotten to service the most important person: me.

(*As mums, the easiest thing to forget is ourselves!*)

‖ PAUSE MOMENT

- Where have you felt burnt out in your day to day? What did it feel like deep within you?

- If you could nurture yourself, what would you do?

- How would that make you feel?

Bring calm in daily

Here are the seven ways I brought calm into my day easily and with little resistance:

- *Mindful warm/hot water consumption on waking:* I would boil the kettle and have a cup of water, either snuggled up in bed or on the verandah at sunrise. The calm comes with being present to the sensation of the water. On my lips, in my mouth and travelling down. It allowed me to begin my day slowly.

- *Prioritising movement for myself:* As you can probably tell from my stories above, fast-paced movement has always been my jam. Yet at this time of needing calm, I had to choose slow and purposeful movement. Running or jogging without a time frame for it. Yoga. Pilates. A stationary bike set up outside so I would get the benefit of the outdoors.

- *Outdoors time:* Realising that rushing through my day was a sure way to burn out was huge for me. Getting outside for my morning ritual or exercise was key to getting more calm in. Just stopping for a quick moment to feel the wind on my skin, the sun on my face and the earth under my feet, even if only when dropping off or picking up the kids up from school, really reconnected my soul.

- *Rest:* Giving myself the permission for middle-of-the-day rest time was essential. Stopping the relentless pursuit of the to-do list, and knowing when enough is enough, as well as lying down and sleeping, was vital.

- *Prioritising early bedtime:* This was a simple shift that meant I moved more towards getting enough sleep. Just a note: in an ideal world, we females would sleep seven to nine hours per night. Now I know that with little people we might get woken up from these sleep times often ... I still do! However, providing the framework for this amount of sleep is really important for cultivating calm. (More on this in the next chapter.)

- *Learning how to breathe again:* Yep, that thing we do every day that keeps us alive is really important for our calm quotient. A simple check-in when we feel the overwhelm, the busy and the stress sneaking in can bring us right back into our calm state.

- *Connecting to my fun and joy:* I am always calmer after I've done something that brings me great joy. Dancing to super loud music, singing at the top of my lungs, having sex ... you know, all the fun stuff!

‖ PAUSE MOMENT

- Which of the seven tools for bringing back calm will work for you today?
- How do you want it to make you feel?

The power of calm in a very un-calm world

It's safe to say that 2020 and 2021 were some of the most unstable years in our modern existence. They have thrown up factors that we didn't even know were a problem in our worlds. The lack of movement in a highly connected world, a virus-pandemic that not only affected health outcomes, but also tested friendships, values and the whole spectrum in between.

This lack of calm created a turbulence that has begun to underpin the human existence (thanks COVID!). It affects our neurology. It can create a trauma response in our system that is similar to that of PTSD and that allows our system to shift towards a fight/flight state more easily and for sustained periods of time.

There has never been a more pertinent time to use these calming tools to soothe our souls. These skills for invoking calm can be cultivated at times of stress — or even just those times when your body perceives something as stressful — so that even if the stress is caused by the outside world, you are able to calm your way out of it.

The stress response is a crazy thing. We explored how it gets embedded into our system in chapter 5. But knowing what you can do, and why, to bring your mama-calm back in is key. It is powerful to consciously be aware of the strength lying within yourself. This calm state is a mama superpower.

The keys to your unstoppable calm are:

- recognising your shift away from calm
- identifying why it has happened
- knowing if you can do something about it now... or whether you need to let it go
- using a calming tool (breathing works great in the moment for me)
- making a choice and reframing the experience
- simply being calm.

The calming tools are cultivated over time. Yes, I still lose it sometimes. The mornings in my house can be crazy. But when I feel that bubbling up inside of me, I stop. I listen within, I try not to react in the moment and I choose calm.

This can be your superpower too!

‖ PAUSE MOMENT

- Where is a common un-calm in your day?
- Which tool will work for you?
- What do you want calm to look like?

Affirmations for a calm motherhood

A super powerful mama can really embrace positive thinking, thoughts and actions through the power of affirmations. Now don't get me wrong... I used to think all of this stuff was super woo-woo! And it definitely has an edge of the woo-woo about it. But it works. Really well.

Along with the positive self-talk, affirmations are one of the greatest ways we can hack our day. I stick them everywhere. On my mirror, in my car, on my screen saver on my phone. The visual reminder of positive self-talk, followed with a loud reminder of my awesomeness when I speak it, is a gamechanger.

The power of affirmations has been explored through social and psychology research. According to psychologist Catherine Moore, affirmations are based on the 'self-affirmation' theory. It is broken into three steps:

1. *Self-identity:* We keep up self-identity with a global narrative or wide-ranging narrative about ourselves. This means we can define success in lots of different ways because we aren't defining ourselves in one fixed way.

2. *It's not just about being perfect:* The theory identifies that our self-identity is adequate in the areas of our personal values, allowing us to be moral, flexible and good.

3. *Self-integrity:* As the affirmations cause us to authentically merit acknowledgement and praise, we maintain our self-integrity. By saying the affirmations, we aren't just hoping to get recognised for it, we *are* who we want to be in that affirmation.

The affirmations for mothers provide us with an avenue to become the person we know we can be. Not just in our mothering, but in our sense of self. Often, as mothers, we can lose that sense of who we are. That sense of who we were before motherhood can be really, really murky. Affirmations are a powerful tool for reflecting on what we could be and what we would like to be, and turning it into a portion of our daily reality.

My affirmations at the moment as I write this are:

- I am strong, capable and connected with my family.

- I choose healthy, life-nourishing foods.

- I am moving like l love myself every damn day!

- I infuse fun into my day.

- I am a wealthy woman.

- I am an author (*hint hint:* Writing a book obvs at the moment so making it about that).

- I listen to the voice inside me because my thoughts are my intuitive self.

II PAUSE MOMENT

- Have you used affirmations in the past?

- What would your top five affirmations be at the moment?

- Where can you stick them, say them and embody them?

Breathing and calm

The final component to thinking like a calm mum is breath work. The most life-changing thing I did was begin to embody breath on a daily basis. It sounds pretty simple, doesn't it? I mean, we all breathe every single day to keep us alive.

I'm going to give you a little backstory here. Unsurprisingly, as a busy, rushing woman, the power of my breath was lost on me. I would rush here, rush there, fit it all in and get my to-do list done, and then I would crash into bed, have a restless sleep and start all over again.

I bet this is a familiar scenario to a few of you too!

When I went through my burnout crisis, I really needed to find a way to hack my vagus nerve and re-establish some calm in my world. I am super blessed to have an amazing friend who teaches calm-inducing breath and yoga for a living. In fact, I work with her in my 6 Week Mama Reset course — which means you can too!: it's the calmly patient Courtney Morrison. She began to teach me some simple ways to really get into this.

They have been life changing for everyone I've shown them to and I'm going to share them with you now.

Before we start, there are a couple of indicators that breathing work may not be for you and that you need to check in with your GP or health professional first: shortness of breath, chest pain, fainting, vomiting or dizziness. All of these indicate that there is something else going on, and a full check-up is vital before beginning these breathing exercises.

Now, on to the main game!

There are two main breathing methods that I want to show you. The first one is a simple box breath.

1. Imagine you have a box in front of your face. It has equal sides.

2. Imagine you go up the left side as you breathe in.

3. As you go across the top you hold the breath in.

4. As you go down the right side you breathe out.

5. As you go across the bottom you hold the breath out.

It's that simple.

I like to do four seconds on each side.

Two cycles of this and I immediately feel centred. Ten rounds and I've totally changed my day.

Then I ask myself, what do I need? Where am I at? What's next here?

And this allows me to get focused on what I need to do now. Just like anything, the more times we do it, the easier it becomes.

II PAUSE MOMENT

- Try a simple box breath pattern for two to five rounds.
- How does it make you feel?
- Where does it make you feel?
- What do you need...like really...after this?

The second breathing technique is a simple yogic breathing pattern that I love called alternate nostril breathing. I'm not a yoga afficionado, but when I discovered this version of Pranayama I was blown away. Of course, the best way to do this is to be guided through the practice in a yoga class or with a breath practitioner, but I've pooled some resources together to support you in starting to investigate this.

When I first do it, I feel a rush towards my third eye. I feel an opening in my awareness of what my brain is perceiving in my outer world. According to an article by researchers Puthige Raghuraj and Shirley Telles in the journal *Applied Psychophysiology and Biofeedback*, the benefits of alternate nostril breathing are:

- nervous system regulation (well ain't that amazing), as the conscious deep breathing regulates your nervous system out of stress and into its parasympathetic or calm response

- lower blood pressure through slowing your heartbeat and, in turn, your blood pressure

- improved breathing if practised consistently because it enables better oxygen flow and you can exhale more oxygen — basically improving lung health

- lowered fear and anxiety due to the lower breathing rate. It's part of the triggering of the stress response in your body. Consistent, slow breathing lowers the feelings of anxiety we get in our system.

Here is a step-by-step guide on how to do alternate nostril breathing:

1. Sit quietly somewhere: it doesn't have to be fancy (I often do it in bed in the mornings).

2. Breathe in. Place your right thumb over your right nostril. Place your second and third fingers along your nose towards the bridge (I like to put them on the third eye region to bring awareness in) and put your ring finger on your left nostril.

3. Open your left nostril by taking pressure off your ring finger and exhale slowly and fully.

4. Block the left nostril with your ring finger, remove your thumb from your right nostril and breathe in from the right side smoothly and continuously.

5. Once you've inhaled completely, exhale through the same side (the right nostril).

6. Block the right nostril, open the left and inhale slowly through this side.

Continue the process. I like to do five cycles. I definitely do this sitting down. Sometimes it brings a lightness and awareness to my body that I wasn't expecting. I love this: it's a connection with myself that I crave in the busy and the rush.

‖ PAUSE MOMENT

- Try doing five rounds of alternate nostril breathing.
- Where do you sense the shift within you?
- How does it make you feel?
- Where could it be powerful for you?

(10)

SLEEP LIKE A MOTHER

Happiness is ... sleeping next to your mother, irrespective of your age.

—Unknown

Sleep. The great big missing link of motherhood for so many of us. I remember while growing up that everyone made jokes about sleeping like a baby as if that was the best thing that could happen in your world. And then my best friend had three babies at once, and I realised it was an absolute shit show at the beginning. I'm sure I'm not alone here.

Sleep as a measure is one of the biggest indicators used in the issue of the 'good vs bad mother' myth that I think we can all personally relate to. There is a lot of societal (think patriarchal) overlay that we are indicated as good or bad mums if we can get our baby or child to sleep according to a particular routine. That if we do things a certain way, according to whatever the expectation is at that point in time, then we are good mums and we have a good baby. Like WTF ... how can we be graded on our perfect mothering dependent on how well our child sleeps!

By the end of this chapter you'll have a great understanding of:
- the importance of sleep for mums
- sleep deprivation and the effect on our health
- values and sleep choices
- the how-to of better mama sleep
- applying the motherhood lens to sleep in the:
  - newborn phase
  - toddler time
  - kid years.

Now, I am a mama who always wanted to do things 'right'. I wanted a child that slept because that meant I was obviously feeding her enough, I was changing her bottom enough, and she was happy and healthy. I fell into the 'good mother myth' that sleep was the perfect indicator of how 'fit' I was to be a mum.

The universe knew I needed a journey through this, most likely to open my eyes, bring me awareness, change my lens of the whole motherhood thing, probably even to prepare me to write this book. And so, my daughter Matilda was born. I've discussed her birth story already, but the nature of her birth (I believe) and the transferred stress she received from moving around internationally when she was a newborn, relayed into a wired-up nerve system that interrupted her sleep. Much as can happen to us. She woke every one to two hours for months.

We tried everything. I thought I was a failure. I read all the books.

The harsh controlled-crying books that advocated letting her cry until she fell asleep—this just wound her up more. The gentle parenting books—which did work but used up so much of my time in resettling her that I literally felt my entire day revolved around making sure

I didn't miss sleep windows and getting her to bed. I tried the demand style of feed and sleep, which did work well, but I was incessantly tired from this.

In reality, she was just trying to find her way in a big new world on the outside instead of on the inside, and together we were feeding into stress cycles. As I've discussed before, in retrospect, the lack of support around me at the time, without my girl and mother community to lean into, was a big part of this stress load. I thought I had it all together, but the struggle was real, and I 100 per cent did not have as much of a handle on it as I thought I did.

It's taken me until recent years though to reflect on how this impacted my sleep in the long term. We know from research that a new mother's lack of sleep quality can lead to depression and anxiety, and according to a meta-analysis on sleep disorders by Yuan Yang and colleagues published in 2020 on the website Frontiers in Psychiatry, there is a prevalence of 67.2 per cent of poor sleep quality in post-partum women.

No thanks!

Working on my sleep has taught me a few things:

- One night of poor sleep is manageable.

- Two nights makes me a bit more cranky.

- A week of poor sleep really does impact my emotions, my inflammation and my resilience on the day-to-day stuff that happens.

My hope in this chapter is that I can help with a few tools, tips, tricks and knowledge to boost your sleep into the realms of awesome (at least a few nights a week anyway) and get your vitality back! Because *booyar!* Vital mums are healthy mums. Healthy mums are connected mums. And we all want that in our world!

‖ PAUSE MOMENT

- What does poor sleep look like for you? When does it happen most often?

- What is your tipping point for lack of sleep? Are you a three- to four-day ninja like me, or are you adapted in the early years and can go for weeks without a catch-up?

- What does great sleep look and feel like for you? How many hours is it?

Sleep deprivation and the effect on our health

According to an article by Eric Suni on the Sleep Foundation website, sleep deprivation occurs in adults when we don't get our seven to nine hours each night. I've spoken to thousands of mums over the years, particularly in the early years, and that amount of sleep is not happening regularly. Unsurprisingly, the Sleep Foundation also tells us that kids require 10 to 12 hours of sleep regularly. If this has triggered feelings of lack and annoyance at yourself, that isn't my intention. I just wanted to bring you the concepts of the ideal amount of sleep.

The term 'sleep deprivation' means not getting enough hours, whereas the term 'sleep deficiency', or 'sleep insufficiency', refers to the quantity and/or the quality of your sleep.

Interestingly, there are three definitions for sleep deprivation. The first one is 'acute sleep deprivation' and this relates to a short period (a few days or less) with a significant reduction in sleep time. In our mum world this might happen when we have a sick child. This time will often last one to six nights, especially if it bounces between siblings where we are up looking after them during the night. Following on from this we have a resumption of normal sleep patterns.

The second definition is 'chronic sleep deprivation'. This is defined by the American Academy of Sleep Medicine as 'curtailed sleep that persists for three months or longer'. I would say that the newborn stages of motherhood can cause chronic sleep deprivation. This definition would also apply to those families that have a child who continues to wake and disrupt once they are past their newborn phase. Frankly, I think in a straw poll of mums in my orbit, that could be upwards of 50 per cent of families at any given time.

The final definition is 'chronic sleep deficiency' or 'insufficient sleep', a combination of sleep deprivation and sleep disruptions occurring throughout the night. This is the category that a lot of us have fallen into during our working-mama load, or lockdown. We stay up later than we should because we need our own time, and then by the time we get to bed we could be facing a maximum of five to six hours of sleep, knowing we will likely be woken during the night too.

Looking through this information was a bit disheartening to me. I don't know about you, but I feel that as mums, we are set up for this to be a hard road. If we then go further to observing the impact it can have on our health, initially it's not too different from many of the things we expect in our early motherhood journey:

- slowed thinking

- reduced attention span

- worsened memory

- poor or risky decision making

- lack of energy

- mood changes.

Once we move into the territory of chronic sleep deprivation, however, a wider variety of health problems crop up. According to the Sleep Foundation website, sleep can impact most of the functioning of the systems in our body, and put us specifically at risk of:

- *cardiovascular disease.* This can manifest as high blood pressure, coronary heart disease, heart attack and stroke.

- *immunodeficiency*. This is a decrease in our body's immune functioning impacted by a lack of sleep.

- *obesity and diabetes*. I'm sure many of you had gestational diabetes in your pregnancy/ies. The regulation of blood sugar is impacted by sleep, which increases the risk of conditions such as diabetes and obesity. If we can treat our sleep disorders, we are more likely to improve glucose metabolism and energy balance.

- *pain*. As we continue to lead an increasingly more sedentary lifestyle and the amount of chronic pain suffering in our society increases, trying to alleviate it through great sleep hygiene could be one of the best key life hacks. There are many elements of sleep that can make pain worse (such as where it occurs) and it can create a tough cycle to navigate.

- *mental health disorders*. The link between sleep and mental health has been known for years. The strong binds between poor sleep and depression, anxiety and bipolar disorder are evident in the literature. As mums, we are more likely to suffer anxiety or depression as a result of lack of sleep, with statistics from PANDA indicating that as many as one in six mums experience at least one, if not both, of these. The impact that the decrease in quality sleep can have on our brain is huge.

- *loneliness*. Yep. How we sleep can affect our connection with others, affecting our sense of loneliness, and this can have huge health repercussions too.

- *response to stress*. It's no surprise to mums here, but when we are in sleep deficit, we respond to low stressors in much the same way as we would respond to high stress if we were well rested. This basically means we get crankier the more we lack sleep. I'm pretty sure we are all walking indicators of the truth behind this.

There is no doubt that our stress load can impact our sleep and that sleep impacts us physically. The flow-through that this can have on our immune health, our perceived stress and our day-to-day life is massive.

As mums, especially if we are working outside of our home, the demands on our day are huge. We are expected to navigate so much with little to no support, and what doesn't get done during the day, gets pushed into the evening or into the following day, just to add to that day's load. So, we stay up late to get things done, we don't sleep enough and we create a state of chronic sleep deprivation for ourselves ... and the cycle continues.

My hope is that by bringing knowledge to how sleep deprivation can impact us, we may add some tools to our day that will make sleep more effective in restoring our system, our health and our mental state. So we can show up as ourselves.

II PAUSE MOMENT

- Where does your sleep suffer? Is there one thing that really gets your sleep off track?
- Is it impacting your health at all that you are aware of?

Values and sleep choices

When we look at changing our sleep patterns and moving away from the societal expectation model we may be clinging to, we can see how sleep and values can be interwoven. As humans, we all go through alterations in our values systems based on where we are at right now.

This is why I will always get my mums to really think about their identity in this space and time (as we did in chapter 6). Who you are, why it matters to you and how that can look on the outside are all valid elements to consider when we're discussing sleep. When we view our sleep requirement through the lens of what is most important to us, maybe it will shift a little and skew towards a change that is more sustainable in the long term. Or at least a recognition that we can choose to do better if we want to.

I have a friend (let's call her MJ) who had health struggles that we couldn't define — there was a missing key. MJ had a busy life. She was working and a single mum looking after the kids 70 per cent of the time. Her kids were super busy, and one of them has an autoimmune disorder, adding to the stress load and management in the day to day. MJ was really struggling with her mental health and her overall zest on the day to day.

Things were feeling hard and she was finding she was drinking a bit much, both alcohol and caffeine. We had a chat about that and she worked on her diet for a good month. I then checked in with her, hoping for some improvement. But for MJ, things felt much the same. She felt she was missing out on her joy points (the end-of-day vino) with absolutely no benefit to how she felt.

So I dug deeper. She was staying up late, until 11 or 12 at night, so she could get all of the jobs done for her family that she hadn't been able to finish during the day. She really wanted to create a sense that she was nailing this single mum life thing. She was so worried about letting her guard down and asking for support, worried that she would look like a failure and weak, that she was driving herself into the ground.

We had a look at her values, and family and health were in there. So we reframed the importance of sleep. We did a time study of her day, and figured out ways to get her some support so she could get some sleep time back. Support came in the shape of getting her mum to help out with running the kids around. She cut back her work hours slightly. She delegated some of the household chores to her kids. She created some 'alcohol-free days' in her week, which allowed her brain to rest a bit better at night. She stopped drinking caffeine after lunch. And she went back to doing some exercise, which improved her mental clarity. Within a month, she felt a lot more like her old self. Welcome back MJ!

I know this isn't a story that we haven't heard before. In fact, we've probably all lived it at various stages. I had to learn to let go of some of the ideals I had around the way my house looked in the mornings, and that some days when I was running out the door I wouldn't leave everything impeccable...and that this was okay. If you've ever seen my live videos, you will know that hasn't changed! Otherwise I would be up until 10 or 11 at night just ticking off the little things I needed to get done.

Sometimes, when it's early enough and my energy is still great, I use the 1 per cent of my day rule to get that one extra job done. Whatever I can get done in 14 minutes and 30 seconds, I will do (you'll recall in chapter 6 that I talked about one per cent of our day being 14.5 minutes). Anything after that waits. Then it becomes down time, calm time, rest time and sleep time.

I had to realise that I was responsible for my own healing; there wasn't anybody else out there who could heal for me, and complaining about things didn't make a difference. It's an inside out kinda job. For me, sleep was a very large component of that shift to healing from the overwhelm, the burnout and the cranky-mum world.

II PAUSE MOMENT

- In what ways do you sabotage your sleep?
- Which value is that linked to in your values list? Can you reframe it so sleep can become important again?

Applying the motherhood lens to sleep

The key to better sleep for all of us is to acknowledge initially that sometimes, if not every night, we can get woken up by the kids and that this will have a bearing on our sleep. We need to allow for that, and increase our sleep time so we can still get the seven to nine hours that we need.

One of the key things we can do as mums is to follow simple guidelines around sleep and how to achieve it. There is a wonderful integrative stress-management and holistic wellness practitioner called Paul Chek. I highly recommend his website, Chek Institute, where he discusses sleep quality and how we can influence it through some very simple actions at the end of the day. There is also a lot of information on the National Institute on Ageing website that will give you ideas on good sleep practices that you can integrate to minimise the effects of aging.

I've combined all of the pertinent information from both websites to provide a thorough viewpoint of how you can help yourself to sleep better — through a motherhood lens, of course:

- *Switch off.* Turn off your phones and devices a few hours before bed, or if you're going to use them, wear blue light reduction glasses — and don't take the devices to bed with you.

- *Have a consistent bed time.* This is a big one for mums. The one thing we can control is the consistency of our bed time, and how we can get our body used to sleeping at a certain time.

- *Cap the caffeine.* Be mindful of caffeine choices and how they affect your sleep patterns. For me, coffee after lunch can really interrupt my sleep. Not the falling asleep part — the waking up at 2 or 3 or 4 am part. I'm pretty sure the coffee doesn't allow my cortisol to drop to the levels it needs to, to encourage that quality deep sleep through the early hours.

- *Avoid late afternoon or evening naps.* These can throw out your sleep routine. This can be tricky if, like me and many mums I know, you had to lie with a child for a day nap and would 'occasionally' nod off. I was all for the middle-of-the-day sleep, however, anything after 3 pm was pretty self-destructive on my quality of sleep at night.

- *Develop a routine around bed.* If you've followed me for a long time, you'll know I use a Shakti acupressure mat as part of my sleep routine, to get my system into calm mode, combined with some breathing techniques and the other things listed here. I just pop it directly on top of the mattress and lie on it on my bed. I fling it off the side of the bed when I'm done, and the wind down from it is epic.

- *Use low light in the evenings.* Paul Chek is really big on this as it helps to support your natural circadian rhythms for the hormones that support sleep. Dim the lounge lights, use the night lights for the kids — or maybe even a salt lamp with its ambient light.

- *Keep your bedroom at a comfortable temperature.* We do this for our kids, but what about for ourselves? I love sleeping with the window open, I really love the breeze and fresh air and it helps regulate my circadian rhythm to the outside temp. But living in Queensland, during the summer I will sometimes use an air-conditioner, as it's just too hot to sleep without it. I have felt guilty about the energy consumption, but it really helps my quality of sleep, and is an important tool for keeping me healthy and my body regulated.

- *Do your exercise at regular times each day.* I'm sure the people who developed this weren't thinking about mums in a very busy stage of life, but I still think that any exercise is better than none. If you can do it close to a particular time each day it will support the hormones and rhythms of your body better.

- *Avoid eating large meals close to bedtime.* Again, if this is the only time of the day you get to have a larger meal, by all means do it. But if you can eat a bit earlier, say at 6 or 7 pm, and go to bed around 9 pm, then at least you've had some digestion time.

- *Avoid alcohol.* It may help you fall asleep faster, but it will consistently wake you during the night due to the sugar.

These are the tips that, on researching, I thought mums could incorporate into their day. Maybe not all of them — definitely not all of them at once — but trying to slowly change up those sleep rhythms and return your sense of self and soul to a calm sleeping environment could be the final piece in your health puzzle.

If you would like a printable resource on sleep, make sure you go to www.workmamalife.com, where you will be able to grab a reminder to stick on your fridge or in your bathroom. Just like affirmations, a little visual reminder can go a super long way.

‖ PAUSE MOMENT

- Which of these sleep recommendations are you already doing?

- Which ones do you think you could incorporate into your day?

- Which ones are laughable in your current situation? (We all have those at different stages of life. I mean, I run an online business, so a few hours of no screens before bed will *never* happen. But 30 minutes is totally achievable.)

The 'how-to' of better mama sleep

Reading through research article after research article, I made some glaringly obvious observations that the research was focused on people who 'work', who 'need down time', or for whom lack of sleep is significantly impacting their health. Research on sleep and the impact of it on mothers is scarce and is, I feel yet again, another indicator of how the patriarchal society expects us to 'just get on with it', even though it may be really detrimental for our health.

I've decided there's no point having a book for mums if I can't give you some specific tools to navigate the actual how-to of sleep. Let's have a look at the practicalities of trying to support our sleep during a variety of stages in our existence as mothers.

First-time mama

This is a tricky season because we face the sudden shift from great (well, until the third trimester at least) pre-parenthood sleep, to waking every one to three hours all night long because a small human depends on us! This is a time in our life where survival is vital. I mean obvs! There are a few simple tricks that I recommend to get you through this time without completely losing your mind:

- *Try to not look at your phone in the middle of the night.* I know it's tempting when you're breastfeeding. It's like a lifesaver, but it also ramps up the 'awake' hormones in your brain, and could make it harder for you to fall back to sleep after feeding and settling.

- *Keep your coffee to a minimum after lunch.* After having my first babe, I couldn't even smell coffee without her not sleeping for days, while with my second I could have that sweet nectar of the gods in the morning and it didn't affect his sleep. If you can function on one cup before lunch, and maybe switch to tea or herbal tea or water in the afternoon, then this can really help your sleep.

- *Move your body.* I know, I know. A broken record, but getting a short walk or small amount of movement into each day will help your sleep quality too.

- *Rest if you need to and are able to.* If you are tired in the daytime, and your baby is sleeping, then forget the dishes, the washing and the million things on your list and just go to sleep. It can be a total gamechanger, and can refill your sleep tank enough to get through the day well. Remember that a whole lot of small stresses can be as bad as a big stress if we are really tired, so try to stop that from becoming a reality for you.

- *Keep the house lights dim in the evenings.* Keep the TV on and engage in conversation, but when you are navigating those frequent wake-ups, sending your brain the go-to-bed signals can create a significant improvement for your hormones.

- *Go to bed when the baby does.* But only if you are not craving mega adult chat time with your partner. Trying to keep to a semi-consistent routine for your bed time is really great for your brain, and we all know we want to support that guy as much as we can!

The toddler years

This is where it can get a bit tricky to navigate your sleep requirements and theirs at the same time. They begin to realise they can get out of bed themselves, they have their own minds and they can push the boundaries around sleep. I've been pretty lucky with the whole going-to-sleep thing with my kids, and they have always been pretty easy to get to sleep. The older one, however, has tested me on the entire staying asleep factor, like FFS: how can an eight year old wake up so often? But I digress... the toddler years are a really important way we can help our body to recalibrate after we have moved through the newborn and infant stages of sleep with our kids.

In the toddler years, I found that sleep routines for the kids were just as important as they were for me — just as in the newborn years, it's vital for us to try to reclaim our sleep patterns. We know that our brain alters during pregnancy and afterwards, meaning that it is highly unlikely we will ever resume our pre-kids sleep habits. We are often wired to wake at the smallest sound from our children, and when they are toddlers this can include them rolling around crazily, coughing, yelling and crying.

What we do have control over, however, is the choices we make in supporting our own sleep habits. Here are some tips for you and your toddler:

- *Have a regular bed time.* Encourage your toddler to go to sleep at a time that suits you (not them). Creating habits that will suit them as they grow up is key at this stage (for all of you).

- *Minimise screen time for toddlers.* This goes for you too. Try having no, or minimal, screen time after 5 pm if you are aiming for a 7 pm bedtime. This will allow your brain (and theirs) to get into calm mode before winding down to sleep. Research tells us that screens ramp up little people's brains, so using them between dinnertime and bedtime, particularly the blue light iPads, can make the wind down to sleep way more difficult.

- *Show them what you expect.* Have a regular bedtime yourself to demonstrate it to them. They will follow your lead, as you are the most important human in their sphere.

- *Figure out what works as a wind-down routine for you.* Is it a 30-minute or a five-minute thing? Are you tired enough that you don't need much support, or is the day getting so hard that you really need the quiet time? Does a 30-minute episode of your favourite TV show, followed by some screen-free time and breath work before bed, work for you? Or just jumping into bed as soon as you can? There is no right or wrong here, just an ability to bring awareness and to figure it out for yourself.

- *Don't be hard on yourself if your bedtime has dramatically shifted.* Having guilt around not making the most out of your day by going to bed as soon as the kids are asleep is not worth it. Sometimes we just need a battery recharge. There are nights where I still hit the hay at 8 pm, and it's magical!

The kid years

The fluidity we can bring into the years once our kids are at school and the freeing up of bedtime routine can make a massive difference to our energy when we are facing the end of the day. Sleep, once the kids are older, is more of a struggle around fitting in all the things that we do, combined with getting the motherhood jobs done and filling our own cup. There is *a lot* that we mums try to fit into our world. This time where kids are in primary school is a great time to begin creating our perfect sleep routine — which, of course, does *not* happen perfectly each day.

As I outlined earlier, there are so many ways we can support our sleep. The key elements are definitely more easily integrated during the kid years, when there is a bit more normality and routine in your sleep world. Here's a recap:

- Switch off and use minimal bright light sources.
- Don't have caffeine after lunch time.
- Journal all the junk out of your head.
- Don't eat and jump straight into bed.
- Exercise regularly.

When we sleep well, we are definitely more linked in with ourselves, our communities and the people we choose to surround ourselves with. My hope is that each mum is able to step into her transformation through honouring what her body needs, not burning the candle at both ends, and allowing herself the space to sit and be calm.

As I spoke about at the beginning of the book, we have times in our life where we have a season of busy, and a season of quiet. Looking at what influences our sleep and changing that can often be best achieved by habit creation when we are in a season of less busy. If you look at this and laugh, however, then maybe less busy isn't on your radar anytime soon. Trust me, I get that.

How about choosing one thing — just one — that could shift sleep for you! You are worth it, Mama!

II PAUSE MOMENT

- Which stage of sleep are you in? What's one thing you can improve tonight?
- What would happen if you didn't burn the candle at both ends? If you chose to honour your intuitive requirement for sleep and health, and allowed your to-do list to roll over?
- How would that transform your life?
- What shift would that be?
- More stress? Less stress?
- Sit and reflect on that now.

Part III
LIFE

Launching your New, Vital Self back into the World

Let's get this show on the road, mama!

You've come so far. I am beyond proud of you! You have the understandings now behind health and how to help yourself. You've stepped through the 5 Pillars of Healthy Motherhood and now it's time to actually make this a reality. Let's bring this joyful, vital *you* back out into the world in a way that doesn't increase your stress load.

As a working mum, I know you have enough going on in your world. I am not in the game of making everything harder for you, so let's discover how to integrate awesomeness back into your life again in simple ways. Don't forget you can go to www.workmamalife.com for all of the free resources you may need to integrate this life changing vitality back into your world!

The message I want to send you in part III is that life is for living, making changes and expressing yourself. How you can make a shift and a change that actually lasts. That is transformative. That allows you to be the woman, the mother, the working mum — any of those labels that you really desire for yourself — in a true way.

It all begins with the transformation pyramid (see chapter 11), which is a framework that we'll use to shift your sense of self and make a long-lasting change.

We're going to look at the 5 Pillars of Healthy Motherhood through the lens of the transformation pyramid. It will take some work, but I'm confident that, through this journey together, you will be able to transform new skills, behaviours and environments in line with your identity and source, allowing you to decrease the overwhelm and reimagine and recreate the life that you as a mum can and should have.

A vital, energetic existence that sits with *you* in your glorious self: a mum who has been able to throw off some overwhelm and fatigue and reclaim her gorgeous, brilliant, vibrant and healthy 'self'!

(11)

THE TRANSFORMATION PYRAMID

How can you create the life you desire — the image that you have of what motherhood should look like — by using the concepts I've shared with you in parts I and II and integrating them seamlessly into this amazing thing we call life?

The answer comes in the form of a wonderful framework that I call 'the transformation pyramid'. It embodies the 5 Pillars of Healthy Motherhood and makes it a heck of a lot easier to achieve the shifts and changes you want to bring into the world for yourself.

I first came across this pyramid thanks to mentors of mine, Dr Don and Brandi McDonald. We have searched high and low for the original creator of the pyramid, but it remains a mystery. If you do know who originally shared this thought bomb, send the reference my way! I would love to acknowledge where it came from.

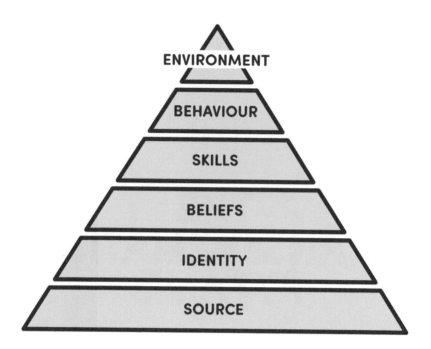

By the end of this chapter you will have learned:

- the levels of the transformation pyramid
- how the levels can integrate into your world.

Bringing joy and vitality back into mum-life through transformation and choice is why we're here. Let's explore the levels of the pyramid, and then integrate it into your world.

Source and Identity

I like to combine the base of the pyramid, Source, with the next level, Identity. The base of any pyramid is the biggest level, the one everything else is stacked on top of, so we need to ensure this level is super strong. We do this through our sense of:

- source
- feeling

- self

- knowing who we are

- what matters to us

- what values are important to us.

For me, having a sense that we're connected to that great big 'whatever' is out there is really important. I grew up in a Christian family, where the sense of source was always assumed as being God, and that formed the next level, identity, as well, because your identity was to be a Christian child. These days I have taken that to a different place. I feel that it's more of a universal presence. Yes, I believe that there is something out there that connects us. I don't know what to call it, or how to label it. I don't know who it is. We can call her God. Mother. Mother Earth.

I don't know who she is, but I'm connected universally through intelligence to her. When I'm tapped into my source, I feel a quiet contentment internally that brings an awareness of who I am and what I stand for. Even in the busyness of my crazy mum work-life, when I can spend a minute connecting back in with my inner intuition — or 'knowing', or whatever it may feel like — I know I'm making better decisions with clarity and calmness.

When I'm more connected in this way, I feel an easier shift to joy and fun. And that my vitality is ticking along on point.

Quantum physics tells me this connection is both internal and external. If you look at the writings of Joe Dispenza (you'll remember me talking about him in chapter 5), you'll find that he discusses the role that our connection with others has in connecting with our bigger self and purpose. When I'm there, I feel a great sense of service to the world. Not just to the concept of the greater world, but also to the mother world, to my family, to my practice members: it's an ability to be connected deeply. This helps to shape my identity.

Knowing that the universe has my back (thanks Gabby Bernstein) connects me to my identity of someone who knows inherently that she is

Ali: a healer, a chiropractor, a mother and a wife. This identity that provides me with the strength to honour that whispering in my soul, that deep-seated sense of helping to change the world one mother at a time. This is Source.

Beliefs

The next level of the transformation pyramid is Beliefs. Beliefs are what you get from your source and your identity. We often start with our beliefs, without first discovering the role that our source — our true nature — provides in setting up that belief structure. We tend to dive into *What do I believe in and what are my values?* without going all the way back to the source of who we are and how this fits. And how this shapes our identity as a human.

My beliefs are that we all have an inherent ability to heal that we often don't acknowledge. That our body is a brilliant entity that has a deeper level of function than we will ever know. That health is really important. That we have everything we need residing inside us. That we are given an ability to connect with others physically and emotionally. We know as humans that, regardless of our distance or closeness to our loved ones, our connection to family (chosen or by birth) is really important for having joy and fun in our lives.

I believe that in an ideal world we can get to a point of communal support for each other. That as mothers we can reach out without fear of judgement — that we can reach out with a deep-seated knowledge that we are strong, and we are capable, and we are resilient, and we are able to ask for help. Especially when we are having days where we don't feel any of those things (which most definitely happens).

Skills

Above Beliefs on the transformation pyramid we find Skills. Skills give us a wonderful toolbox full of things to transform our world. If I'd written this book two or three years ago, I probably would have started at this Skills level and missed the foundational elements of Source, Identity and Beliefs. But that would have been wrong because we start with our source, we determine our identity and then we get our belief structure. And only after that do we put the skills in place to actually help the change and the choices happen. We create a skillset around ourselves that gives us the support and ability to change things as we need to.

Skills are really important in making our world into the scenario that we want it to be, to give us the ability to cope with change and transformation as required, and allow us to fit into the world in a way that doesn't drag us down and create an overwhelming heaviness.

Skills are individual. In the following chapters, I'll share some of mine with you. My skillset is communication with others through the written or spoken word. It is my healing hands, and it is science-based neurological knowledge and my ability to disseminate it down to understandable chunks. It is being able to take that brain information and make it into words that people can understand easily and with no confusion. My skills are warm hugs and great coffee. And connection with my kids. I love my skills.

Those skills support my beliefs because I think the more knowledge we give mums and the togetherness we create through communication and channels, the more our abilities to connect with each other and regain that community mentality will grow. And that's our skills around our mothering practice, which is separate from us as mothers in our motherhood — which is a really important delineation to understand.

Learning how we can lean into our skills—how we can use them to interpret our source and to choose transformative behaviours for ourselves — is a key way we can unlock the overwhelm and get rid of it for good. The skill of mothering (the tasks and day to day actions), are not what defines us as mothers, or what defines motherhood. As soon as we have a child we are a mother. We are expressing our version of motherhood. How this plays out isn't dependent on any perceived skill level — this is purely the action of mothering.

Behaviour

As I touched on above, if we have the skills and the knowledge, then we go up to the next level, where we actually start making changes to our life. We've upgraded or finally begun to understand our source, we've worked on our beliefs and we now know our skills, so we can integrate these into daily or weekly behaviours. This shift in behaviour will allow us to connect with that deeper sense of identity and source. Our inner 'why'.

Behaviour shifting, for me, is going to bed early after getting up early. I know my brain works best in the morning so writing this book, for example, supports my skillset of writing, which in turn supports getting this book out on time, which then supports my identity of being someone who supports mothers. This connects me back to Source because I feel most connected early in the morning.

That's an example of behaviour shifting to warrant a skill to match my beliefs and my identity to get to Source, but I wouldn't have known why that behaviour was important if I hadn't been able to track it down to the four levels that came before. As mums, when we are time poor, we are stressed and overwhelmed, and we often dive deeply into the behaviour change. But it doesn't stick. We aren't able to make a long-lasting change because we haven't been able to understand the *why* behind it. This is where the pyramid of transformation really comes into its own.

Another example of behaviour shifting is health. Health is an important belief; it's part of my identity. Being healthy is important to me, and it is also a core part of who I am. I know that when I'm at my healthiest I connect better to Source. I can drop in. I can meditate. I can feel that calm, connected centredness that I need — even in the crazy, even in the busy, I can feel it.

A behaviour that I know supports that for me is eating healthy food and prioritising finding time to move my body. The behaviour shift happens to support the other four levels. I get up early, I do some bike-riding,

I move my body, I eat a great breakfast. And those behaviour patterns set me up for a great and healthy day.

Environment

This leads to the tip of the pyramid, which is Environment. Sometimes we can begin our transformation journey with the environment and turn our pyramid upside down. We try to make change happen and alter our life. We'll start with Environment and Behaviour and decide that we might get to Source later on, if it ever comes to that. But this deep work is the hard part that generates the shift inside all of us.

The environment component is where there's a behaviour shift. We need to support ourselves with the people around us. I've already introduced the concept of the five most important people in our lives — or the five people we spend the most time with — being the ones who are going to shift us. The people who most influence us in our behaviours: those things that we do every day to make a life worth living. The questions we need to ask are, *Is my environment supporting me for healthy choices? Is my environment conducive to going for a walk? Is my environment conducive to not living in a state of anxiety or stress due to a domestic situation?* All of these elements — and more — make up our environment.

✳✳✳

There you have it! The transformation pyramid in its essence.

This pyramid completely embodies the shift and change that we can get as we reclaim our life for ourselves. We've learned so much through our exploration of the 5 Pillars of Healthy Motherhood, and now we will progress through how to throw away things that don't serve us, maybe add in some that do, and wholeheartedly embody this healthy and heartful mother existence.

(12)

THRIVE WITH YOUR VILLAGE

As mums who work, who are trying to do everything—including striving for a change point in their life—there is nothing more powerful than surrounding yourself with a collective of awesome women on the same path.

Not only can our village be our biggest cheerleaders and support, but they can also be the group of peeps who help us clarify and live out our values. The beginning of my 6 Week Mama Reset and Unf*ck Motherhood movement highlighted to me how much a collective vision between mum's can allow a shift to happen.

I want to start by disclosing one of the myths about villages... that they have to be big. Our village, our community, the people we serve, who serve us and who we surround ourselves with can be small or large. There is no right or wrong way to exist among your collective of women.

> By the end of this chapter you will have learned:
> - why your village matters (a recap)
> - how to use your village to help get rid of burnout
> - how to support your brain with your village
> - how to integrate village into your day and thrive again!

Let me give you an example of how we are often told, even subliminally, that our village doesn't matter, or that it is frivolous. We know that a lot of the men in our world work hard. I live in a town where there is a large number of blue collar workers doing 12 to 14-hour days of labour-based employment, and my understanding, from speaking with lots of the mums, is that the boys need their outlet and they get it without really needing to determine how it fits into the family structure.

I think it's essential for men to have 'men time'. It's part of their human condition that they connect in a masculine energy way with each other away from the work environment. It may be out fishing or watching footy or drinking beer or having a BBQ or running a marathon or building a car or going to the movies. There's no right or wrong, but men definitely need their 'man-time'.

What we need as women, though, is an understanding that we also crave 'village' time in our beautiful, feminine energy space. And women's village time shouldn't involve women catching up while also playing with or looking after children (because sometimes the quality in that is tough to find). Or sneaking village time into a 10-minute coffee at work (which, of course, can be fabulous, but how much can you connect in 10 minutes?). Or doing it on your only day off... when you just need to nap or rest or get on top of that ever-present to-do list. What we need is to have a society that has minimal judgement around women needing this connection time. A society that understands that we aren't selfish mums for expecting to be honoured in our neurology of connection with our peeps.

A while back, I was having my hair cut and listening in on conversations happening around me. I've engaged in some beautiful discussions with amazing women by doing this. Ha ha. These wonderful women were discussing how they had to ask permission to get a night out. Not just the logistics of organising it, but that it really had to be a granted reason to get out the door. Unpacking this as a patriarchal over-reach could take up an entire book, but let's just say this isn't a fair situation.

We can also feel a level of anxiety when we have time away from our kids. This may be expressed as mum-guilt — that feeling that you can't have fun or do things without the family because if you were the best mum possible, then you would 100 per cent of the time want to be with them. Maybe there is worry that things might go wrong, that your partner won't look after the kids properly. Maybe it's your first time away from them, or you're breastfeeding and not sure if they will need milk on demand.

These emotions aren't wrong; they are actually 100 per cent normal for mums the world over. A large part of developing ease in our motherhood journey is being cognisant that we can feel these feelings, and that they are part of the normal human existence.

(***Self-acceptance for who we are right now in this moment is transformative.***)

Who wouldn't be worried about leaving their child/ren for the first time? Or even the tenth or twentieth time? Stepping away from our kids can be tough and leave us guilt ridden.

You know what is great though? It's when you know who you are and what your values systems look like, you have your village and you get to knuckle down with them on these very topics when you're feeling the feels. Your village is part of developing an ease and recognition of 'self' within your motherhood journey. Having them around you is great.

Let's explore how to thrive within our village, and what this might look like for you. Busy working mum, stay-at-home mum. However it sits ... let's get that shift happening.

‖ PAUSE MOMENT

- When was the last time you were able to hang out with the person/people in your village?
- What's great about hanging out with your peeps?

Burnout and village

As busy working mums, we know that one of the first things we stop doing when life gets tough and relentless, is hanging out with our village. I mean, have you ever had those times where you are so stressed, the thought of discussing it with anybody brings you to the point of tears or exhaustion? I have!

I remember being in South Korea, living the expat life. I was concurrently writing and running an online program for chiropractors to upskill their communication and assessment techniques when working with children, raising two humans and supporting my husband while he was working six days a week. On top of that, we were dealing with family stuff back in Australia, and it was a load to carry. There were days where I felt I couldn't keep on doing everything, and I couldn't see a way out of the quagmire.

I knew I had gotten myself into this mess because I took on the online work even though I'd been gifted the chance to be a mum full time. At the time I didn't understand my self-worth or my values systems enough to realise that my online program was an important element of who I was and my identity. So I was blindly trying to do all of these things and slowly burning myself up from the inside out.

Now there are two things to unpack here ...

One is that I had this vision of my self-worth that explained away my feelings, and that the overwhelm and exhaustion were of my own making, so I couldn't complain. It was a problem — and not honouring what I was doing daily as important for my *soul* was fuelling my concerns of overwhelm and fatigue. What would it mean if, as women, we were drawn to the things we love to do for our *soul* purpose, and were openly supported in this?

What if this enabled us to feel free knowing we have a level of support that enables us to try hard and achieve. The exhaustion and fatigue would be gone. If we had our village of women around us who had our back, who we could lean on in these crazy times, that would be life changing.

Which brings me to the second thing. That I didn't want to call anybody to help me, or enlist my girlfriends, because I had crafted such a strong mask and persona that I was the lady who got shit done and managed to have it all.

> **I didn't have the strength in my honesty to be imperfect. I didn't have the means to want to bring that up.**

Now, thankfully, my village recognised this, and they stepped in. We organised a girls' night out. We had a few more play dates and I got my son into an extra three hours per week of playgroup so I could have some breathing space. I leaned into my husband, who supported me by giving me some kid-free time in the evenings to get some extra work done.

The biggest block I found to this was that I didn't want to put anybody out by asking for support. I knew that everyone was busy, and that they all had their own stuff going on. Yet I'd forgotten the pleasure I gained in supporting other women. How supporting other mums when they had stuff to get done really made my soul feel complete and my heart happy. I was worried that my race to burnout might impact other people's race to burnout. I'd forgotten that we were so interconnected that one of the best ways to look after myself was to support others and seek that same support. And when I did, that's where the soul nourishing and on-fire moments happened.

The race to burnout as a working mum can be epically quick if we don't have that village to back us up. That community that understands us, and allows us to fly and soar. That recognises our identity and who we are at the Source level, supports us in honouring our beliefs (even if they don't quite fit theirs) and helps to provide us the environments we need to be our best 'self'. Not just in the work environment, but in our *soul* and our sense of *self*.

II PAUSE MOMENT

- When have you felt utterly supported by your village?
- What did that look like? What did it feel like?
- Where have you supported other members of your village? How did this make you feel? How awesome was it to support somebody else?

Your brain, with community, will thrive

Our brains are wired for connection. I touched on this earlier in the book, but here's a quick recap. As outlined by Matthew Lieberman in his book *Social*, we are profoundly shaped by our social environment, and a jarring social interaction can be as painful for us as physical pain. We are shaped by the people we surround ourselves with, and the motivational landscape of our environment can drive how well our brain functions. In other words, as humans we are social beings. Our brains absolutely love connecting with others, and if we have a troubled interaction, it can be as painful for our brain as a painful injury is for our physical body. In other words, being around people can be great for us!

Lieberman discusses in his book how we continually scan our social interactions with those around us to drive our behaviours so we can fit in better. We try to, in essence, mindread each other, so we can predict what others are feeling or thinking and alter our responses appropriately. I know that when I'm at a party, I'll scan the peeps around me and I'll try to sense who is on a wavelength like mine. It's subconscious, but I'm sure this is how I ended up drawn to those women I discussed in the first part of the book.

I mean, if that isn't a strong indicator for tribe in our world, I don't know what is. Social elements of life create a thriving community. As mums, we can look to the concept that cavewomen were working mums too. An article on the US website Moms maintains that nearly 50 per cent of female workers have children under the age of 18, which is a huge shift from 50+ years ago with statistics telling us that only 34 per cent of mothers with kids worked then. There is also a lot of discussion around the inability of women to do the work of men due to competing requirements on their time and concentration. Recent discoveries by archaeologists found that mothers have always worked to provide for their families. In fact, the highly skilled big animal hunters of the caveman era were comprised of 30 to 50 per cent females, indicating a much more equitable division of tasks even back in the hunter-gatherer days.

So, as mums, with the changes that happen in our brain as we move through pregnancy and motherhood, we can acknowledge that we have an altered sense of connection. Yet our social element is vital for human existence. It can form part of our source or identity, even though, historically, we had been assured that wasn't the case.

I remember for years, when doing my values lists, I was always drawn to joy and fun. Yet I felt that to be an exceptional human that was not the way to go. There was no space for joy and fun for me. As I've gotten older, I've discovered that my brain is wired to respond best to social cues. That my ability to avoid overwhelm and fatigue is to regularly top up my social brain. Maybe this is why I rely on interactions in my daily life as a chiropractor, or in the playground with other mums. Or dinners, or lunches, or running dates.

However it comes at me, being able to *thrive* is reliant on regular check-ins with my village.

Thriving looks different to all of us.

Thriving is defined as 'prosperous and growing: flourishing'.

When, as working mums, we are in flow, and in our health and vitality space, we can't help but flourish with those around us. As working mums, we get stagnant and stale when we are unable to thrive and flourish. Recognition that a large part of that is connection with our village and our social interaction with others is super important for our brain to work effectively.

II PAUSE MOMENT

- When do you thrive? What does it feel like?
- What does it look like?
- How does your brain feel when you are thriving and flourishing?

Integrating village into our day to day

We know now how important our community is for our health. We know how important our community is for our success. We know that if we are strong about our values, we can make everything happen that we desire. We know all of this.

Making it happen can be the next tricky thing, but I know you've got this, Mama. The balance between self-love, self-worth, family, social time and your work life can be all consuming. But the ability to balance well, and flux and change depending on what season of life you are in, is imperative. Working with 100s of mums in my online course world, I have found that completing a simple time study, which you can download for free at www.workmamalife.com, can help decrease the overwhelm that we can feel when we first contemplate this change.

Community is defined as 'a group of people living in the same place or having a particular characteristic in common. The condition of sharing or having certain attitudes and interests in common'. Our community is vital for us to succeed in this thing called life. Incorporating it into regular life without creating extra stress is the hard part.

Incorporating community may look like:

- a weekly lunch/dinner/brekky/coffee with a girlfriend
- a phone-a-friend tree for when you need extra support, or that messenger group where you all send stupid memes, as well as the serious stuff when you need it
- a regular date night with your partner
- a professional mentor group/coach who can support your ideals while understanding your motherhood journey
- integration of a village with the health ideals you are hoping to acquire (running club, cooking club, yoga class, meditation workshop)
- playgroups and play dates where the kids are taken care of by other people and you can socialise.

The list for community integration is endless, and finding one or two that work regularly for you is a great way to reconnect. Finding a way to bond with my fellow mums and to keep my sense of self-worth together while I was leading a busy life was vital. I made time for it when it was connected to my ideals, my source and my identity. If I was constantly asked to do things that didn't fit with that, even subconsciously, I didn't enjoy it and it became a chore.

Use your body as a barometer for where your village fits. Your body has an amazing ability to know what is best for you. By tapping into it, even when it is about village and choices of social interactions — a seemingly external element of our health and wellbeing — we can gain a massive improvement in connection status. Asking for help and support doesn't make you weak, and when you get that support around you, you can really get an integrated village-style life going on.

We exist in concentric circles of connectivity. The five people in our super inner circle, including our partner, may flux and shift to the next circle out, which comprises 10 to 20 people, and then out to a max of 150 people in our strong acquaintance circle. For me, the colleagues I see at seminars — and who I absolutely love spending time with because we have similar values and ideals — are my outer circle. My girlfriends — who I have grown with through university or afterwards — are my next circle in. And closest are my husband and my handful of best friends.

Depending on where I'm at in life, there has been some flux between the two inner circles, but integrating them and knowing where to lean for support has enabled me to integrate this village continually at various stages. The times I didn't integrate my village was when I wasn't valuing my own self and I didn't understand why seeking it out was important.

Integrating community successfully required understanding my values and self-worth, and knowing who to connect well with. I know you've got this, Mama, and you can find your village. It may just take some practice.

‖ PAUSE MOMENT

- Who is in your three circles? If you could lean in on anyone right now, who would it be?

- What integrated tribe practices would you like to include in your day/week/month?

(13)

FAMILY FUN AND A NEW YOU

Stand in your own light to bring a brightness and lightness to others.

Navigating the shift to a vital, joyful and healthy motherhood and life is the bomb-shizzle. It's not without some challenges but we can often end up being a beacon of fun and change for our family, much like a lighthouse. So let's get ready for our shining moments. Let's have a look at how we can smooth the entry of new-mum into the old family unit without ruffling too many feathers.

After reading this chapter, you should come away knowing:

- the tools to navigate any family push back
- what it feels like to stand in your own light
- how to acknowledge your emotions: the mum edition
- about environmental integration and the new you
- how to get your family and your shiny new 'self' happening.

Any big change can throw a cat among the pigeons. It can unravel a pattern that has been occurring in your dynamic for years, and it can create a lot of turmoil. I've seen it firsthand. In fact, I've lived it myself. I remember when I decided I wanted things to be a certain way with my health, and how that meant changing things at home. There's nothing I write about in this book that I haven't explored for you first. So here's my story, and a few of the hot tips I learned along the way.

I was recovering from burnout and decided I wanted to have a pattern to my day to allow some restoration of my nerve system: some calm functioning that would enable me to support myself and heal. The choices I made involved journaling, lights low, lots of rest, calm movement and minimal stimulants in my day (caffeine, sugar, booze, etc).

It was a big shift.

I was consciously moving away from heavy exercise mode, which my body was telling me was not okay at this time because it was taking me days to recover from each workout. And I was consciously moving away from the stimulants that made me feel like I could do it all. Yet, the expectation from my kids was that I would be hill running out the front as they walked the dog, or running beside them as they scooted. The expectation I felt from my husband (that wasn't actually true) was that I wasn't exercising enough. I'm not sure what 'enough' was perceived as being, but my internal narrative was telling me I had to exercise to look a certain way. Understanding that getting my body back to its pre-motherhood size and shape was *not* indicative of how healthy I was on the inside, was in fact, a massive shift.

Over time, the more quiet and calm in the house, the altered light ... all of this led to a decrease in overstimulation, improved sleep and better cortisol levels — and the rest of the fambam got on board too. The kids took up swinging in a hammock while reading at times when they might otherwise have opted for screens. There was more natural movement towards nature play. But it took some time. And there was a journey of inclusion for the whole family that we had to work through to make it happen for us.

Standing in our own choices can be a ride. We have all the feels, all the questions, both externally and internally, that we have to navigate and move through. I've done it. I know you can too. Let's dive into the conversation around this.

Navigating the family push back

Now that you are beginning to choose a different way forward, embracing the 5 Pillars of Healthy Motherhood and using your understanding of Source from the transformation pyramid and who you are to make your shift, you may be experiencing a little bit of push back. Integrating a new you into your family and your environment can be a bit tricky at times, so let's navigate this together.

How can you overcome push back from the other members of the family as you integrate this shift? You will be feeling different, and showing up differently in your day to day. Up until this point we've discussed owning our stories, and being aware of what this will look like for us and how we can choose our own motherhood adventure.

It might be because:

- food choices in the house are suddenly different
- you want to get outside and move more instead of watching TV
- you are going to bed earlier
- you aren't drinking as much booze in the evenings (which may be something you used to do with your partner).

I mean, I'm cranky at myself sometimes when I begin to choose something different, so why wouldn't my kids and husband be annoyed if I suddenly altered their diets to a healthier one? Navigating the tricky emotions and the big feelings that could come up around our new choices is a large part of the change.

I was researching how some of the most prominent people in our world recommend making change and I came across a 2015 blog by Brené Brown titled 'Own our story. Change the story', in which she discusses how writing a brave new ending in our personal lives means three things. For me, this can be choices around our 'self' and our health, and our vitality and who we are, as much as it is around discussing hurt and shame. I'll share Brené's top three tips below, and then we'll expand on them with the lens of motherhood and family at the forefront of our minds.

1. Hurt feelings within families can turn into anger, bitterness and loneliness so we must talk about them — even if we're feeling tired or we don't want to. We can't simply ignore them.

2. If we want to write a new story and (in Brené's words) 'pass that legacy of emotional honesty and health down to our children', we have to accept and verbalise any family history of addiction and mental health issues.

3. To learn and grow, we have to own our failures and mistakes. It's uncomfortable and hard, but it's a brave move. And it will unleash creativity and innovation.

Looking at this, how could the first tip show up in the family and in motherhood? Your spouse or partner, or even a child, may be bitter or angry if they feel your choices could be negatively impacting them. Does what you are doing impact them? Maybe a change in diet is making their body scream out for what they are no longer allowed to eat. Maybe the decrease in screen time is aggravating them. Maybe you stepping into your light and making healthier choices is creating some shame for them around the choices they make.

Does this mean that mothers shouldn't make those choices?

They should do what's best for the family, even if the perception is that the old way is the best way forward. I mean, let's be frank. I've raged plenty when I've changed how I've done things. My body has ached and screamed for the sugar and the caffeine, and it was willpower and values reflection that got me through it. It's pretty normal to ride this wave.

In our family, there was a lot of acknowledgement of feelings and discussions around *Why?* There were also times when I gave the kids an ice-cream to stop their rage. I ain't no perfect mother. But the slow shift towards wholefoods and calm over time really paid off. Sometimes ripping off the bandaid is a great option. And maybe it is for us too. But if we are choosing to integrate shift into our family, and it's our choice not theirs, some gentleness can be great too.

This plays perfectly into the second tip on Brené's list. We know that emotional honesty about how it feels when we make big changes can be the catalyst for shift in a family. This book isn't about changing psychology, but it is about navigating change and shift. In a specific family unit, there may be a history of trying to make change that doesn't stick, or a history that there is only one way to be healthy, and it's the opposite of these more vitalistic choices you are making. Acknowledging, discussing, sitting down and speaking through what it could look like if we all made the shift together ... this is the emotional heavy work. You might need support through this. Or you might not. Give yourself and your family members the space to explore how that will look and how they will show up for you and cheerlead you on your journey. This can also be a great way to turn around that mental heaviness.

When you begin to put yourself first again and recognise your self-worth, a level of engagement needs to occur internally to give you the strength to have these conversations.

The most important of the three tips is the third one: navigating the family push back by acknowledging when you don't do as well as you could have. Ask for support and let them know what was hard about it. We can't ignore hurt feelings in the family. Explain the process. Having honest conversations about the best bits and the toughest bits is really important. This also opens up conversations for when our kids or our partner are navigating challenges and acknowledging tough things about how it's okay to learn and grow from these situations.

Honestly making a conscious conversation about the changes to make is the first step in navigating the family push back. And maybe your family will be ringside cheerleading you on. Maybe with the understanding of the background and what you are wanting to achieve, they will be there shouting you on from the sidelines the whole way!

Over my journey, I found the re-introduction of 'me' time the hardest part. Discussing why it is important to you, how you choose to try and make it work for the other people in your house and how it is your time. That's why it's great for honesty to play such a big role in family conversations. The openness doesn't always translate to acceptance, but giving yourself and your brain the chance to get in there and make a change is super effective.

I would love to be everybody's cheerleader as you move through your 5 Pillars of Healthy Motherhood. I would love to see you soar and fly. You may be like me, and go gung-ho early, and you may need a partner who is accountable to get the right choices happening on those days when you really want to slip back into the old ways. But the best thing is learning how to be your own cheerleader!

It can be incredibly daunting to have the conversations around the change you are bringing. Reflection on your 'why' is really important if you feel there may be push back. These conversations don't mean that there will be absolutely no concern about the changes, but having a strength and understanding in your convictions can make it easier.

II PAUSE MOMENT

- Write down the changes you are going to choose to make in your world.
- Why are they important to you?
- How do they fit into your values systems?
- How do you see them fitting into your family's way of life?

Standing in your own light

One of the hardest parts of developing our sense of self in this new world is knowing what this will feel like: *How will I be this person? Who is the new healthy mama? Is that an identity I can relate to?*

Yes, we can have a logical understanding of what this could look like for us in the real world. But knowing the feelings of what to expect — and how to actually know when we are in our 'zone' of motherhood and how this can then integrate into family — this is one of the hardest things.

So let's work through this a bit more. Rediscovering feelings of who we are away from our family, and then trying to figure out what that morphs into when we are immersed in our family environment, is a big part of owning ourselves when we are with our loved ones. There are still going to be times when we feel we are disconnected from ourselves or our family, we aren't being our best self and we are just a cranky mo-fo. Don't get too disheartened.

This is all normal — it's part of the human existence. We ebb and flow. We exist in calm states and in busy ones. The ability to recognise, to switch and to move in accordance with what is required is one of the best indicators of a state of balance in our 'self'. It's not that we don't ever experience those emotions it's that we can recognise them, acknowledge them and let them guide us to where we need to focus.

Are we feeling this way because we're incongruent with our values?

Are we feeling this way because we're tired and not nourishing our body well?

Are we feeling this way because we're strongly in our power and nothing can shake us?

Are we feeling this way because we currently have a lot of patriarchal pressure in the space we're filling?

Are we feeling this way just because we are? There's no specific reason for it — it just *is*?

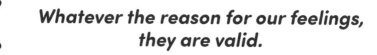

(**Whatever the reason for our feelings, they are valid.**)

I find journaling my feelings works for me. Also chatting to my husband or my best friends about why I may be feeling that way. And sometimes, I just need a nap.

Acknowledging emotions: the mum edition

I'm no expert on mental health (there is a world of psychology out there to equip you with tools to support yourself, so if you feel this upcoming section might be too much for you, seeking that level of professional advice is highly recommended).

What I share with you below is information collated from a number of reputable sites that I have used to create a proforma for leaning into our feelings — for accepting them. I've placed a motherhood lens on this so we can begin to see things from our own sense of self.

From here, we will explore how this could look within the family unit.

To begin with, we are going to look at how to identify and acknowledge our emotions. From the verywellmind.com website, there is a three-step process of emotion identification. It suggests you pick an emotion you can feel that isn't overwhelming you.

(1) Identify the emotion

First, we want to identify what emotion you are feeling right now. If you are feeling more than one, choose the one that is easiest to identify.

Once you have identified it, sit and think about how it is showing up for you both physically and in your thoughts. If you can name the emotion, write it down.

(2) Get some space

Now let's try to create some distance between you and the emotion. If you feel safe doing so, close your eyes and imagine that the emotion is a full arm's length in front of you — just out of reach. Try to put it away from yourself so you can examine it.

(3) Give the emotion a form

Now that you have placed your emotion outside yourself, ask yourself some questions about it, imagining it to be tangible. What size is it? What shape is it? What colour is it?

As you imagine it with its size, shape and colour, watch it for a while and recognise it for what it is. When you are ready, let it return inside you.

Reflection

Once you've completed the exercise, reflect on how this experience felt for you. When you placed that emotion out in front of you, how did it change? Did the space give you the opportunity to find a different perspective? What was the size, shape and colour of your emotion? At the end of the exercise, did the emotion feel different?

This exercise is powerful for recognising emotions and feelings. Let's adapt it to you in the essence of who you are. We've worked hard at determining what your source is, who you are and what matters to you. From here, with the skills that we have shared through part II of the book, you've crafted a concept of the mum you want to be. That amazing mama who is striving to avoid burnout, kick patriarchy to the curb, work well, mum well and live well.

Discovering your new self

Recognition of what it may feel like as a mum to inhabit this new and exciting space is a big thing.

Let's run through the exercise we just learned, to give you that beautiful nuanced sense of what discovering your new 'self' could feel like. Instead of focusing on the emotion, let's create in our mind's eye a picture of our new self. Let's really envisage what this could look, feel and sense like.

(1) Identify who you are

Sit back and relax. Get a bit comfy. Close your eyes. How does the concept of a new you feel? What feeling does it bring up? Grab that feeling. Maybe it's excitement. Maybe it's nervousness, anxiety or fear. Maybe it's courage and strength — whichever one is easiest for you to feel at this point in time when you are imagining your 'self'.

(2) Get some space from your 'self'

Now that you've recognised this feeling, let's build some space from it. With your eyes still closed, imagine that the feeling is out in front of you. You can see it. You know it's there. You can sense it. It fills you with the feels, but it is separate from you.

(3) Give your new 'self' some form

If this feeling had a look to it, what would it be? Does it have a colour? A shape? A size? Does it look like you? A new version of yourself? Is it you as you imagined you would be? What feeling are you sharing out? What is the essence of this shape, colour and size?

Once you've recognised this feeling of the new you, welcome it back into your 'self'. How does this feel as it settles back in? Is it filling you up from the inside out? Is it a new you? Is it a stronger you?

Reflect on this as an individual

How did this exercise make you feel on reflection? What form did you give to your feeling? Who were you in that moment? What was the strongest feeling for your renewed sense of self? Are there other reflections that you need to make in order to feel that sense of renewed strength and understanding of who you are in your 'self'.

Reflect on this in your family unit

Reflecting on this as part of the family unit, do the same feelings come up? Do you want to redo this exercise as part of the family unit? Are there blocks? Is it easy?

How can you feel the seamless integration of a new you into your family? With this exercise in your toolkit, hopefully you have the space to be able to pause for a moment.

II PAUSE MOMENT

- How did this step-through of emotions and your new 'self' make you feel?

- Where can you feel a roadblock for integration coming up?

- Where can you sense a freedom of expression first showing up in your motherhood and family unit?

Environment integration and the new you

Taking time to imagine and feel who you may be, and how that may fit into your family, can provide you with some amazing nudges. Nudges on where you may need to shift your environment, or even the things you do within your family. Nudges that may work towards creating harmony between your sense of yourself in the family unit, and who you are internally.

When we are making lots of new changes there can be some easy shifts. For example, if you are looking at upping your nourishment game, getting back on track with your eating and allowing yourself the freedom to choose wholefoods, then creating an environment around you that supports these actions is essential.

Chuck out (or donate if applicable) the food that doesn't serve you (or your family). Make a list and stick to it at the shops so you can begin replacing unsupporting nourishment with supporting food. Make a menu plan that will suit the kids as well as yourself. Nothing derails healthy eating concepts quicker than the thought of and actions behind having to prepare more than one meal for each sitting.

I've been there, cooking up to three meals per night. It is soul-destroying. I mean, all those bloody dishes, and all the thought processes about timing it so everything happens at the same time. No thanks. I'm supposed to be helping my family eat cleaner and easier, not make more work and overwhelm.

If you are looking at exercising more, then how can that fit into what is considered your 'normal' day to day. How can you make it fun? Can you incorporate it into a time you would normally spend doing something else you really want to stop doing? Can you do it in the morning? Over lunchtime? Naptime? After work, before you head home? (This has never happened for me, but I know there are plenty of working mums who manage to fit it in.)

For me, as my kids have grown older and my workload outside of the home has increased, I have progressively had to find weird ways to make this work. I used to be the early morning exercise girl. The spike of cortisol and the happy hormones set me up for the day. As mindset coach Ben Crowe would say, 'Win the morning, win the day'.

Now, however, in our family dynamic, my husband can only get his fitness in at 5 am, which means I am at home with the kiddos. This has allowed me to fluctuate my workouts. And during the COVID restrictions, they definitely weren't prioritised.

Sometimes I'm super motivated doing sunrise yoga or HIIT workouts on my verandah. Sometimes I'm not.

As I write this, I'm finding time in my week on a Monday and Friday after school drop-off to do boxing classes. On Wednesdays I run and/or bike-ride, and then on the weekend I try to sneak something else in too. The biggest shift for our family now that the kids are older, is that we can exercise with them. We can make it fun and sustainable. Sure, it's not as sweaty as pre-kids, but it's still fun and it's connection: a double win!

The environment for thinking and calm is the one I struggle to alter the most within my family unit. It's the one that I seem unable to get happening with the kids or my husband around. You see, we live in a small house. A really small house. I don't have a space to set up as a meditation corner, with salt lamps and crystals and so on. I'd love that. But it's just not in my life right now. So I have to do it on the go. With this in mind, I've made the strategies I've chosen to share with you in this book easy to adapt to lots of different situations. We can breathe slowly in the car, in bed or lying beside our child/ren. We can listen to meditations and have calming thoughts when we are doing the housework, or if the kids are asleep. We can integrate calm into our day.

Some years ago, I was talking to a busy mum who was embarking on a new meditation journey. She was desperately trying to get herself into a morning meditation routine. She loved the concept that Joe Dispenza had of getting up super early and meditating to get the day set up right. However, with kids who woke through the night and a busy work environment to tend to, she was mindful of burnout coming from these best of intentions. So she got up at a manageable time for her and sat in her loungeroom with a guided YouTube meditation playing on the TV. With the kids creating chaos around her, she would breathe and sit in the moment. Interestingly, at the beginning, the kids would draw her out with fighting, with demands ... you know, kid stuff. Yet slowly, over a few weeks, they would sometimes get involved with her. Sit quietly beside her, fall into breath with her or just quietly amuse themselves. Of course, there were mornings where the wheels fell off, but it was a manageable practice that she felt set up her day well.

By incorporating meditation into her day, this mum worked within her own circumstances, which was essential because she didn't want to add to her to-do list. The shift was tangible for her and her kids, and allowed her to begin her day from that calm space.

Sleep and environment is an easy hack to incorporate into your busy mum-world. As I outlined in chapter 10, there are so many ways we can set ourselves up for a better version of sleep. The hardest thing can be kicking those old habits to the curb. In what ways can you influence your environment to make a good night's sleep a reality? The conscious choices we can bring to our end of day to alter our sleep behaviours are many and varied. Incorporating better sleep for the entire family is giving to everyone — especially when you all have that rush element in the day to day to get everything done.

I've found that keeping the lights low at the end of the day is essential. Minimising the kids' TV and screen time after school makes a huge difference to them ... and on reflection, trying really hard to do that for myself is massive too. I now charge my phone outside the bedroom, set up a timer for the WiFi in the house and put all the devices onto aeroplane mode so they aren't syncing information during the night. All these little things add up.

But the biggest environment shift for me, as I mentioned in chapter 10, was getting a Shakti acupressure mat, which I place on my mattress for 10 to 20 minutes when I first get into bed at night. It, combined with my breathing, calms my soul and encourages deep, restful sleep. I pop it onto the mattress and when I've finished, I tuck it away between the side of my bed and the bedside table. That's how I shifted my environment to support the need that I had to reconnect with myself, allow my body to heal from the burnout and embrace healthy sleep again.

Environment changes within the family unit involve you deciding what matters, and then seeing how to incorporate it with least amount of stress. I can guarantee there will be some teething elements to it, but in the medium term you will feel the ease of the environment matching those concepts of who you are, what matters and how you are choosing to heal and direct your energy into your 'self'.

‖ PAUSE MOMENT

- Where can you easily alter your environment to support your new goals and your new family connection?

- Which part of your environment already supports you?

- What's the one thing you will choose to change tomorrow with the family? How can you get them on board?

Your family and your shiny new self

This leads us to how your ideal family scenario would look, feel, sense and *be* after you express your new, aware, conscious and healthy self. The best way to make it happen is to have a clear vision of what it will look like.

Earlier in the book, I touched on the concepts of *be*, *do* and *have*. You've discovered who you want to be, and things you need to do in order to have the healthy motherhood you desire. Applying these concepts with consideration of the family environment can be a big change that takes time, but is ever so rewarding.

If you want to *be* a certain way, how can your family support you to do this? In an ideal world, what support structures would be in place, how would your change help them and how can they help you change?

If you find yourself running into the ground with an endless to-do list, how can you cross 'dump', 'delegate' and 'do' off that list? Is there a significant other you can delegate to or a paid support person? This comes from a position of privilege, and I fully acknowledge this. I've spoken with mums who enlist their village tribe to support them in their big passion through childcare, home care and connection. Maybe this is your ideal family scenario. This is your chance to dive into the ideal of what that would look like.

Your family love you. You love your family.

It's okay to love yourself too.

Expressing yourself within the family scenario will lead you to be strong. So imagine what that would look and feel like for you. You can *not* control what the rest of the family will do. You can *not* control any push back they may have. You can work with them, you can workshop it, you can discuss what could work and what doesn't work — but, ultimately, you are in charge of you. They're not.

Here's how I work, continually, on creating the ideal 'you' in my family:

- Creating on paper a vision of what a harmonious family environment would look like with the kids and my husband involved is a crucial step in making it happen.

- Sitting down and being open with my family about my needs and desires. How can I let teamwork make the dreamwork?

- Allow them opportunities each week to say what has and hasn't worked for them. And me the opportunity to explore this too.

- Focus on myself, my goals and my mindset daily.

- Remember that I look after *me*, and then I look after them.

The vision that I hold for each of you is that you can figure out how to navigate these, stand in your truth, give your brain a break from doing everything, and be honest with yourself and your loved ones about who you are, what you need and how, together, you can make shift happen!

(14)

YOUR JOYFUL AND VITAL SELF IN A BIG WORLD

I choose joy, fun and vitality, health and commitment to self!

We've knuckled down on showing up for ourselves, in our village and in our family. Woot Woot! We are so there! Now it's about bringing that new and joyful self of yours into the big wide world.

Showing up consistently with the mask of not being burnt out, of choosing health and our 'self' can be tricky. I mean, seriously, wearing that mask all the time represents a busy mum waiting for a crash to come.

The world is set up for us to be relentlessly busy. When did it become a badge of honour to answer the age-old question, 'How you doing?' with 'Yeah, great, been busy ... So busy, just ticking along ... Busy ... You know, mum-life busy.'

No wonder we are burnt out, overwhelmed, tired and fatigued *all the time*. I'll never tire of calling out that the biggest issue facing mums is the relentless expectation from a patriarchally designed society to work as if you don't parent, and parent as if you don't work (thank you Annabelle Crabb for putting this so eloquently).

> In this chapter we will explore and honour:
> - showing up and owning your self-worth
> - being a bold beacon for yourself
> - the ease that comes with regularly 'showing up'.

When I was trying to integrate my 'new, improved' version of me into the world around me, it was a tough struggle at times. The world wasn't set up to allow me to express myself fully, to honour that there were days when I needed rest and days when I needed to be doing the things that had to get done. My internal judgement about choosing rest instead of hustle and grind was, I think, the biggest hurdle to overcome.

I probably needed to overcome more self-talk around my understanding of my self-worth and why it mattered that I showed up as me in all my flaws and awesomeness. Having grown up with a mum who only sat down to rest if rest involved producing something — stitching, reading, family histories (she would totally agree with me here) — there were heaps of layers to break down around what makes a rested mum. Self-worth is a massive component of understanding why you matter, and particularly how rest might play out in helping your brain, yourself, your family ... all the things that are high on our values list.

According to positivepsychology.com, self-worth is defined as valuing yourself, and having a sense of self-value means that you are worthy. Broadly speaking, the alteration in our sense of self when we step from our career or pre-kids mode into mum mode can cause a large shift in our self-worth. So how do we find out why we are worthy? How do we value ourselves more? How do we define our self-worth now?

I'm so excited to figure all of this out with you.

Determining your self-worth

Merriam-Webster defines self-worth as 'a feeling that you are a good person who deserves to be treated with respect'. This sounds pretty good to me. Just like Aretha, a bit of respect doesn't go astray. When I reflect, I can see how there have been times where I most definitely have fallen out of the self-worth frame of mind while navigating this big, fat mothering journey.

The aspect that hits home most to me — and triggers me a bit, if I'm being honest — is being treated with respect. On reflection, those early days of mothering are a minefield of lack of respect. I mean, since when does a newborn baby respect anyone's sleep requirements? Ha ha. In all seriousness though, we get so used to leaning in to the needs of these little people around us that we forget how to lean in to our own needs.

In 1976, two researchers, Martin Covington and Richard Beery, published a textbook called *Self-worth and school learning* that expounded the now commonly held principles of self-worth theory. This theory identifies four main elements to the self-worth model:

- ability

- effort

- performance

- self-worth.

Looking at this, it can be pretty easy to recognise how working mums in particular can identify with decreased self-worth — and how striving for self-recognition could easily drive us towards burnout. Let's break this down together.

Ability

As a mum in the throes of all the mothering things, looking at how we determine if we have the ability to mother 'well' and then combining this with our shift back into the workforce can be trying. In a world navigating the pandemic, there was a global decrease in support for mums. I know that locally, due to social distancing, they stopped all of the face-to-face check-ups for babies, and the support classes for new mums — and the loss of village was immense. Yet this also parlayed into a loss in confidence in our ability to mother. Especially for all the first-time mums out there, this lack of confidence can be quite soul-destroying.

Effort

Nobody can deny that mums put all of their effort into their kids. There isn't a mum out there who hasn't sat up all night google searching why their baby isn't sleeping well; or how they could do this, that or the other better. When effort isn't defined by a perceptible shift in outcome, however — as it most likely would have been in the workplace — our self-worth diminishes. Measuring effort in motherhood is like measuring the sand in a kid's sieve at the beach. Really bloody hard.

Performance

There are no performance measures for motherhood.

Let's say it all together again: there are no performance measures for motherhood. Mothering is best seen as a journey and a constant learning process of shift and change. In our patriarchal society, we are defined by how well we do things, with measures and reports and all of that KPI stuff. In school it is how good our grades are, or how well we compete in sports carnivals. Once we leave school, it might be how well we perform at uni, landing that new job, or the accolades we receive. Maybe our performance is connected to how well we keep our weight down or have the willpower to do things a certain way.

Society drives us to believe that we are worthy when we do things well. But how the f*ck do we do that in motherhood?

Is measuring how well our child sleeps an indicator of our performance? *No!*

Is measuring how early our child develops their gross motor skills a measure of our performance? *No!*

Is measuring our ability to keep a clean house while raising a child, and possibly working, a measure of our performance? *No!*

There is no true way to measure the performance in your mothering, so drop it like it's hot!

Self-worth

This is truly the wrap-up of the other three elements. The concept that there is a way we can measure our worth based on achievements is really not suited to motherhood.

While searching for a more modern take on self-worth — minus the overtones of achievement as the only characteristic — I stumbled across Stephanie Jade Wong, a writer for the 'Shine' app. In her article '13 things that don't determine your self-worth', there were a few things that really jumped out at me as being super relevant for mums:

1. *Your to-do list.* The never-ending task list for mothers that is utterly relentless. Don't let how much of your to-do list you've ticked off define your self-worth.

2. *Your appearance.* Getting back to your pre-baby body is not a measure of self-worth. If you want to do it, awesome, go for it. But if you know that's not your journey right now, that's cool too!

3. *How many friends you have.* When you begin to navigate your world in matrescence, your friendship groups can change. Counting how many friends you have can be fraught with feelings of insufficiency. It's better to instead look at having even one or two friends you count on when you need them and who treat you well — and vice versa.

Now that we have this overview of what self-worth is, and what it isn't, let's look at how we can influence our own self-worth. Referring again to the writings from positivepsychology.com (because these experts are so amazing), there are different ways to rediscover your self-worth. If you are really struggling with this, seeking professional advice would be best. However, here is a simplified version of how to make it work:

- Increase your self-understanding of how important you are. Reflect on how others see you, the things you do that are great, and the areas where you might question or doubt yourself. Coming into this journey by honouring who you are is a perfect first step. (I love to journal on this one.)

- Accept the good, the bad and the ugly around the things you question about yourself — this is really important.

- Write down ways you can love yourself and how you can show yourself the compassion that you most likely throw like confetti at other people.

- Remind yourself regularly of your self-worth. You are not on this Earth to please other people, and you are in control of how you feel about yourself. Step into your power and ask yourself, *How would my best self respond to this?* and then do it. The more you do it, the stronger you become.

- Remember that *you* are the boss of *you*! There is nobody else who has the personal power to change things as much as you do.

Stepping into our self-worth as mums is huge and it is a powerful step into the light of showing up as us in the world. Rediscovering the power that resides within us and the power of choice is huge — and it's a massive part of the self-realisation of how we can have an amazing motherhood, work life and sense of *self*.

‖ PAUSE MOMENT

- What do you currently value as the most worthy part of your *self*?

- What are five great things about your *self*? (Mine are my hair, laughter, zest for life, cocktail-making ability and passion for my work.)

- In your ideal world, how would you represent your self-worth? How great are *you*? (Write it down, sister. Let it fly across the page and imagine that nobody is going to read it; it's just by you for *you*!)

Bold beacons

Being a bold beacon for yourself can be pretty daunting. I don't mean that you have to jump out there and sparkle (although I'm pretty sure if you know me IRL you'll see a whole lotta sparkle), but what it does mean is that we can honestly know who we are, and be that person.

Naturally, there are days where our sparkle may be a little dimmed. Those days where we've not slept, or we just don't feel all the vibes. They happen and they are natural and normal. Just like many of you, there are days where I wake up and I feel like I've slept on a bed of nails. Days where I can really feel my frustration with the world leaching out of my soul before I jump out of bed to face it. There was one significant day recently where I just didn't want to parent. The thought of navigating shower, clothes, lunchboxes, my own lunchbox, driving to school, being 'nice' at work all day, and then coming home to do everything that needed to be done was just too much. I got up, tried to move my body and got interrupted by the kids for what felt like 1000 times. I was shitty. I yelled. I stomped. I acted like a spoilt teenager.

I went and sat down in my room. I breathed. I had a shower and I put on some tunes. I made myself scrambled eggs and a coffee. I knew if I showed up to my practice like this, the universe would energetically cancel heaps of my patients during the day (yep, she's always listening and does this). She didn't, and the day turned around. In fact, interestingly, I had three conversations with mums experiencing a similar day to me. And I could guide them on choices to change it up.

Being able to recognise that I wasn't my beacon self and using the skills to change my internal environment in order to change my external environment was key. It would have been so easy to stomp through my day. I've done that before. And by the time I get to the end of the day I'm tired and angry. My body aches and I try to go to bed early but that doesn't happen so easily. (You know those nights where you are lying in bed full of regrets for the day?)

Recognising that you matter and that your self-worth and strength in choices can create a bold beacon future for yourself is a massive step. As a working mum, the energy it will take at the start may sometimes be hard to muster. Stopping that negative internal chatter when it begins to come up is really important. Recognising that it isn't all rainbows and unicorns, and that the hard work matters, and gets easier over time: that's how we become bold beacons!

And those days where we jump out of bed with the sun shining straight up from our crown chakra, well aren't they the bees knees! I totally love them. I own them! And I try to rock 'em when they happen!

‖ PAUSE MOMENT

- How do your days of less sparkle show up?
- What does your bold beacon day look like?
- What do you do to bring back the shine?

Honouring *you* gets easier

You are worth the effort of getting rid of burnout, overwhelm and fatigue and sparkling from the outside in.

Keep it fun.

Find a way to make it joyful.

Shout it and sing it when you have the urge.

Overcoming the burnout of trying to do everything that doesn't reside well within your values systems is a massive task. Burnout happens when we try to do too much and it goes against our true self. Integrating *you* into the world is definitely easier when you understand yourself more deeply.

Starting with something easy allows you to get that sense of achievement that we all neurologically crave through our reward centres. These are the parts of the brain that send out all the happy chemicals when we do something well. It's like giving yourself a giant pat on the back. That's why our kids beam from the inside when we acknowledge them!

Once we start getting that effect in our brain, it then craves more of it. For me, it's like when I decide to eat really cleanly to help my body function better. I start with the easiest thing for me, which is always sugar.

Stopping sugar gives me an immediate sense of *I can do this*. It takes me about two days, and I feel confident that I'm on my way to getting the greatest results. Once I've done this level of easy, I then move on to the hard... stopping coffee. Each year I'll do a few weeks to a few months caffeine free. I find it reduces my fatigue massively and allows me to reset my overwhelm factor. As with anything hard, the first five days are difficult to navigate, but once I get there, my internal sense of strength and courage is huge. My brain's reward centres give me a massive clap on the back, and I feel empowered because I've made such a great choice for myself.

From here, I often launch into a change-up of my movement routine, or a new job task. Something that takes that level of confidence in myself to get it done. It's really interesting how honouring myself allows my sense of self to be strong enough, to be brave and courageous, to allow me to choose to do new things, or things that have been hard and on my list for ages. It completely reframes my self-worth factors, and I really feel that beacon self internally.

My hope for you is that there is a simple skill step that is transferable to the work place, outside of the home and inside of the home that you can stick to and that will allow your inner sparkle to shine out! That one thing that once you achieve it helps you feel glorious and in control.

Strong,

Brave,

Resilient

YOU!

II PAUSE MOMENT

- What one thing can you do to create yourself as a beacon in the outside world?
- Where have your burnout and values been a struggle in the past?
- How can you *honour you*?

(15)

SELFISH MOTHERHOOD AND WHY YOU MATTER

When there's more light emanating from you, there's no room for darkness.

Being selfish during motherhood isn't selfish — it's bloody survival!

What selfish looks like could be throwing away the mum-guilt, or acknowledging that the paths that bring us to motherhood are different from what we have been told and expected. There are so many wise people in the world who tell us that self-care isn't selfish. Pretty much this whole book is about a journey to self-care that will bring you back to vitality, health and self. Much like my program, The 6-week Mama Reset Program, where we focus on bringing back the health and heart to motherhood. It's perfectly selfish motherhood!

It's about living in the space of your own light and feeding those gorgeous flames that burn within you, so you can move out of the darkness of your situation and embrace *you*. In the previous chapter we discussed mama self-worth and how having it can help with the massive shift to knowing why you matter in the world. Taking this sense of self-worth out into the big wide world can improve your confidence immensely.

So now you are confident in who you are and why you are so important. Let's look at this in the frame of mum-guilt, self-care and mothering when we are working peeps.

You will come away from this chapter with some strong concepts and actions around:

- mum-guilt
- the 'good vs bad mum' analogy
- the difference between selfishness and narcissism
- affirmations for a perfectly selfish motherhood.

The concept of being a bad mum if you work too much and don't prioritise your tiny little human and, as they grow up, your big humans is quite pervasive in today's society. While I strongly feel that during COVID there was an increasing recognition and understanding of the work mothers do, there hasn't been much of a shift in the overarching expectations from society on mothers in the workplace. We saw in the previous chapter how the mum-guilt phenomenon of mothers being expected to work as if we don't have children, and to parent as if we don't have a job, has created stress for mums.

Knowing who you are and why who you are matters is key to having a perfect level of selfishness in motherhood. A level of selfishness that enables you to have self-care without guilt. That's what I'm talking about: owning your self-worth and embracing the importance of it is a daily actionable task. Let me give you an example.

This morning I woke up. I knew I didn't want to cook brekky and that it is food shopping day, so the pantry is minimally stocked. I have the privilege of being able to order food from a local café so, after asking all the members of the household what they wanted — at least five times (ha ha) — I got the order and rang it through.

I quickly sorted and whacked on a darks load in the wash. Had a quick shower and remembered to pop some moisturiser on (total win moment).

Then I realised that I had to get all the bikes off my husband's car rack so I could drive it to the café (because the way it was parked in our driveway meant that there was no way I could get my own car out without doing this). He comes out and we start unpacking and unloading from our adventure the day before. Jump in the car, head to the café, grab brekky, next stop to grab newspapers, head back home. Historically I perceived this little 10-minute adventure as my 'me-time' in the day which, ironically, only served to support my belief that my 'me-time' was something to fit between other activities, rather than to prioritise it as a standalone requriement for the health of me as a mum.

Next, shepherd everyone to the outdoor table, get the knives and forks, listen to the door slam as the kids go in and out to get their special knives, sit down and eat. Bees fly around. Clean up the plates, head inside. Think I might get some time now.

Realise the washing has finished, swap it over, put the next load on, then hang up the first load. Sit down with husband to chat about superannuation — we often have these sorts of chats over coffee. Figure out I need to get to the house next door (my office space currently) to start writing this chapter... Look at kitchen on the way out, wash the dishes, put on dishwasher before I go.

Collect my things and head over to the house. Coffee in hand. Sit down at computer.

Take 10 big breaths. I have space, but I don't classify it as 'me time' because I'm working. I know you get this. That work time is the substitute for me time — but this roundabout is how we get to the burnout and ill-health stages. It's taken a whole lotta work to separate those two. What about you? Is your work time perceived as your me time?

The difference between selfishness and narcissism

Conversations around narcissism have escalated over the past few years. I've seen this through the lens of domestic violence, especially narcissistic abuse from spouses. If you want to dive into this, you can find some interesting research articles in the reference section for this chapter at the back of the book. I'm going to skip this minefield today.

Within maternal narcissism, there is a subtype called covert or vulnerable narcissism. This is different from the largely understood grandiose narcissism, where outwardly everything is about them. Yes, if you search you can find plenty of articles about narcissistic mothers trying to recreate themselves and the things they retrospectively hoped for themselves in their children. Research tells us this results in neglect and psychological trauma for the kids when they are treated in that way. This is a horrendous outcome of narcissism in motherhood.

In a 2018 *GoodTherapy* article by Katherine Fabrizio, she outlines how a mother with 'traits of covert narcissism may appear, on the surface, to be self-effacing and self-sacrificing'. However, due to the heavy involvement in *all* of the child's activities, it is the 'needs of the mother rather than the child, that are the central driving force in the relationship'. I've popped a link to the article in the references, but here are a few key points about where narcissism may be apparent at various ages (the article specifically addresses mother–daughter issues):

- *Toddler and preschool years:* As the daughter exerts independence, the mum uses punishment and shame to stop the 'rebelliousness'.

- *Adolescence:* The mum involves herself in all of her daughter's friendships. She may also exert her dominance around appearance, clothing and social circles.

- *Marriage:* The mum decides on the wedding plans and they are often mother–daughter decisions rather than couple ones.

This kind of paints a picture. I know when I read this, there were a few elements that I recognised. It brought up ideas around the 'Good Mother' and the 'Good Daughter' complexes that, if you're like me, you probably kinda just fell into for a little while. This level of narcissism, while not always recognisable initially, is pretty distinctly different from the traditional caring mother, and hopefully, your own good self.

A selfish mother, on the other hand, is one who — in my view, at least, and through this lens of motherhood as a construct and you as an individual — is able to prioritise herself as a necessary conduit to show up best for her family and community. A mother who is perfectly selfish. Who honours self-care and self-awareness to bring the best to her mothering. Selfish is defined by the Oxford dictionary as 'lacking consideration for other people: concerned chiefly with one's own personal profit or pleasure'.

> *I would like to offer up that in our modern world, with expectations placed so highly on mothers to do everything, a little bit of a selfish life is essential for our own survival.*

It's unlikely — and I would contest if you have made it this far into this book — that you lack consideration for others while being selfish. But to be gloriously selfish is life-affirming. The idea that we still matter when we are undergoing this motherhood gig is oft forgotten.

Aiming to find a balance between your own needs, so that your cup runs over, rather than functioning on half-empty all the time, is where the space of selfishness comes into its own. I remember observing mothers, prior to having my own children, take time to be on their own. They may have come into my practice alone, or gone for a solo haircut or just a walk and a ponder at the beach. These acts of superb alone time were essential for them.

But in retrospect, I think I was judging them for wanting to have this time. Yet, at that time in my life, I didn't understand the continual to-do lists racing through their heads, the time demands of their little people, and their continual striving to allow a relationship with their significant other to not falter, and hopefully thrive a little.

Reflecting on my own parenting journey, there are definitely times where I have felt this judgement. Whether it was my own story that I had to get rid of, the story that if I was taking time away I was not a great mum (more on mum-guilt in a sec) or if it was perceived from others, there was judgement there. The Good Daughter complex, where we are striving to fulfil the role of a good daughter as we think society portrays it, and then the shift of this into the Good Mother role, is a minefield for judgement creation. Recognising that the driving force behind our actions is trying to fulfil someone else's perception of what makes a good mum is one of the greatest shifts we can make towards a gloriously selfish motherhood.

Consciously bringing awareness into my days that the selfish elements allow me to be a better human and prioritise some self-care is vital for my balance in this life gig. Hopefully by just having this conversation on paper, it gives you a bit of strength to choose one small 'selfish' thing to do today.

❚❚ PAUSE MOMENT

- Where in your life have you felt selfish?
- Was this actually self-care dressed up as guilt perhaps?

Mum-guilt and motherhood cups

Learning how to be strong in the sanctity of our own superpowers and how they need to be charged up is a massive guilt hurdle to jump over. The cups of motherhood that we have to continually fill with new volume and liquidity are pretty damn big. We need to look at how we can do this and keep our status of healthy, vibrant, joyful and vital mum intact.

Assuming you have now thrown away (or at least recognised and released) any guilt or stories you may have about your self-worth and how looking after you isn't important, let's take this awareness and look at our mama cups. (Not our mama jugs: you can keep them in your shirt.)

The cup analogy of self-care isn't a new one. As mums, there are lots of ways we can explore filling our cups. I personally like to look at neurology (brain function) as a bunch of buckets, but we could look at it as cups too. In neurology, we look at how the nervous system perceives things, such as pain, when the bucket runneth over and the brain identifies that the pain pathway has been triggered. When we examine the role that filling cups has in motherhood, it's a bit like a leaky bucket.

We have the cup, but if we don't continually fill it up, people and circumstances keep coming and scooping out of it, or cutting little microscopic holes in the bottom. So our cups get depleted. Our cups are pretty much the same as the 5 Pillars of Healthy Motherhood:

1. nourish

2. move

3. think and calm

4. sleep

5. connect.

How these cups need filling will differ depending on where you are in your life, in your day, in your headspace. If there is one cup that feels particularly empty, focus on that one for a week and see what happens. I like to do a Sunday evening reflective practice where I think about my cups, where they are sitting and what I need to focus on for the week.

For instance, as I sit here today, I really feel that my nourishment cup hasn't been great lately. A few too many wheels of brie cheese, and not enough vegetables have entered this amazing body of mine. So I'll spend five minutes writing out my vitamin, movement and nourishment plan for the week. It will be printed and put on the fridge. I may also write some affirmations down (we'll talk about affirmations next) and pop them on the kitchen cupboards, just to give me that little extra rev up.

It's interesting, when we bring intention and focus to filling our cups up, how we can choose to change small things to make a difference. During my week, I intentionally move with the kids. There are also times during the week when the kids watch me work out at the gym. Then there's intentional cup filling where we've organised to hang out with friends (social cup filling, anybody?). The roundabout of guilt and choices is real for all mums. Our ability to navigate this is a key to recovering from burnout mode into nurture/selfish/self-care mode and creating ongoing choices that are sustainable and real for us right now.

‖ PAUSE MOMENT

- Has self-care filled a cup that you've needed to fill? A social cup? A love cup? A health cup?
- Which cup is running high at the moment?
- Which cup is feeling really depleted?
- How are you going to choose something different this week to fill a cup?
- Does this bring up a feeling of guilt for you? Journal this and uncover where it may come from, and how you can identify it and kick it into the curb moving forward.

Affirmations of a perfectly selfish motherhood

Perfectly Selfish Motherhood.

It's that part of us that yearns for permission from ourselves, our partners, our communities, our workplaces and our greater society to be able to honour those quiet voices living inside us with the choices we know we need to make.

I bring to this table of confusion and questioning about how can we do it … drum roll, please … Affirmations. I know I've touched on them earlier, but they really are a powerful way to set the tone for your subconscious and allow it to become a part of your reality. I feel it is one of the key ways the mums in The 6-week Mama Reset Program make big changes. Affirmations provide a voice for those inner thoughts that perhaps you have felt aren't ready to get out into the world just yet. Those little brain thoughts that are 'too good to be true'. Those realisms that you may not have understood how to make real, or how to picture. Affirmations are a super powerful way to tell ourselves what we most desperately need to hear, and the more we use them, the more we make them a reality.

It all sounds a bit woowoo — but there is a special kinda magic in the woowoo! And I can't wait to make it a reality for you.

The affirmations that I most commonly use are listed on the next page. Sometimes I like to record them so I can hear myself saying them. I then repeat them out loud to myself. I often write them on my mirror in my bedroom, or stick them on sticky notes on my dashboard in the car. I've popped them on screensavers on my phone and I've even written them on the bathroom mirror.

They are a great tool that we can use with our kids too. Giving my kids the gift of an internal dialogue of strength, courage and love as they jump out of the car at school is a blessing that we need to bestow if we can. The topsy turvy, high stress world that we have been experiencing over the past few years has, it seems, passed on to our kids. We see it in their eyes and souls each day. We see it in the alarming increase in mental health concerns in our children. A selfish motherhood isn't just for us, it's for them too!

When we show up as our best self, we are able to give them the best of ourselves, and that can only provide a great benchmark for them to grow and develop from. To model off. To learn from. To add into their subconscious.

But back to the affirmations. There is no right or wrong. There is only what feels right for you. I strongly encourage you to write some that give you that inner 'yes' feeling when you say them out loud — that's when we know they are right for us. Here are a few of mine.

I am a strong and courageous woman.

I am a great mum.

I value myself.

I deserve to be me.

I deserve nourishment.

I deserve movement.

I deserve to love myself.

I am loved.

I am Love.

I am loving.

‖ PAUSE MOMENT

- How do you think affirmations could play out in your perfectly selfish motherhood?
- What are five you can start with today?

(16)

THE WRAP-UP: YOUR MOTHERHOOD REVIVAL PLAN

Creating a revolution in our motherhood starts with us flowing out into the world like a ripple effect onto a sea of calm!

Revolutionising your motherhood choices and your health starts with you. You can choose how to show up, what this is going to look like for you and how you are going to frame this for the generations after you. By working through this book, you have learned that there are so many external factors driving you to act, behave and mother in the ways that you do. That the expectations of doing can drive you to an early death.

This final chapter is all about re-energising the newly discovered you in the big world. It's the game plan for change. For my online course, The 6-week Mama Reset Program, I developed a framework that you can use to provide you with some simple reminders of the choices you make and how they can create a shift.

I called this framework the Motherhood Revival Plan.

(By the end of this chapter you will have your very own Motherhood Revival Plan!)

It's short and sharp and gives you the tools to revolutionise your world, reclaim that health and vitality and restore balance from the chaos and dishevelment we all experienced during COVID.

This plan will help you to reconnect your health and heart back into your motherhood. Make sure you download your free worksheet from www.workmamalife.com so you can print it out as many times as you like and get your choices happening.

As busy mums, we all need a plan. A plan that we can bring into the world for ourselves. This plan is going to wrap up all the elements you have learned and processed throughout the book in a short, sharp and succinct way.

I don't expect each of you who have got this far to do everything at once. In fact, I'd highly encourage you not to. I've found that making a substantial shift is something best done slowly, rather than going headfirst into changing *everything* right at the start.

Working through this plan results in a beautiful list that you can refer back to when you're ready. Or you can copy it and stick it up somewhere in your house so you have a visual reference. I love doing this. It's much like my affirmations plastered all over my bedroom mirror so I get a reminder every day of my self-love. You can choose what is going to make a shift for you using actionable reminders.

(You deserve an awesome motherhood. The affirmation I would love you to have at the outset here is: 'I am committed to honouring my beautiful self, how important I am and that I matter.')

My Motherhood Revival Plan

Okay, let's do this! It's as simple as answering the following questions. You can write your answers on the lines here in the book or wherever suits you. Just make sure you can refer to your answers easily any time you want to.

My core values are:

_____

_____

_____

My internal beacon shines when I do this:

_____

_____

_____

I am going to find a collective and nurture it by:

_____

_____

_____

I choose to eat and drink to support myself by:

_____

_____

_____

I choose to exercise by:

_____

_____

_____

I choose to nurture my brain by:

_____

_____

_____

I choose to find calm in my day by:

_____

_____

_____

I add fun and joy to my day by:

_____

_____

_____

I choose a mama sleep experience that focuses on:

_____

_____

_____

I deserve to honour my new self because:

_____

_____

_____

I will look at my work–life balance through:

_____

_____

_____

Things to remember

You, gorgeous mama, who are working hard to keep yourself healthy, recover from burnout, overwhelm and fatigue and regain some zest and vitality... you are worth it!

There is nothing harder than learning how to reprioritise yourself when you are shifting and changing. You will 100 per cent fail in some of the choices you make. But you are strong. You can get up and try again.

There hasn't been a healing journey I've taken where I haven't ended up falling off the wagon at some point. Maybe I was trying to decrease my toxic load... but someone got me a coffee. Or I really wanted to eat more wholefoods... but the appeal of a wrap was greater than the much healthier salad.

You know what I mean. Sometimes human nature is just that: human nature. Sometimes my hormones are stronger than my willpower, and the magnesium hit of chocolate beats any strong intention I may have. Or I really need that super strong black tea after lunch so I can get my focus back.

What I have learned the most is not to see this as a sign that the rest of the day is ruined, or that I can't start again. Not wiping off a whole day, or week, when all I need to do is make a small, mindful shift is the key to making the change. And being aware of consciously choosing that thing in that moment because it is the right thing to do is just that: a choice.

You are worthy of choosing your own life.

Small steps is how lasting change happens.

You can make your motherhood revival exactly how you want to!

CONCLUSION

We've reached the end of our journey together, and what an absolute ride. My hope is that you leave this space feeling the empowerment that I was hoping for. The empowerment to making shifts and changes in your world away from the burnout and the overwhelm. Away from the fatigue and the frustrations.

My hope is that you have discovered a sense of inner strength that you didn't otherwise feel. Make sure you go and check out The 6-Week Mama Reset Program if you want more support on this journey.

Or maybe you just want to print out your revival plan. You can go to www.workmamalife.com for all of the printables.

I also hope that you've been able to embrace your own ability to choose joy, health and vitality.

I know that 2020 and 2021 massively shifted the load on mums the world over. The brilliance and gorgeousness that still resides within you hasn't changed though. That innate sense of who you are and your ability to shine bright like the amazing diamond that you are.

This reimagined, thriving motherhood allows you to be bold within the precious life that you live.

You are worth it, Mama. You can heal and grow and shift and change!

I love you!

Get out there and love yourself too!

APPENDIX: RECIPES

Hello beautiful Work Mama Lifers!

Here is a collection of my favourite, generally easy, nourishing recipes that we love in our house. At the beginning of each week, I sit down and think about what we will eat and how to make it work easily.

The first step is to get my shopping list sorted, do the shop (I love online, but often don't quite make it happen) and then start cooking. I've divided the recipes into brekky, lunch, dinner and snacks, and I've added in a few of my own creations. Sorry there are no pics. I'm not great at those. I am great at using leftovers, though. 😊

Breakfast

Overnight oats

www.superhealthykids.com/recipes/basic-overnight-oats-recipe

These overnight oats are great. I'll often make up a big batch on a Sunday night and this gets us through the first few mornings of the week.

This recipe is super simple, and you can add or take away whatever you want. I normally add in some yoghurt, frozen/fresh berries and a drizzle of honey. To increase the protein count, I also stir through some collagen in the morning, as protein is really essential for our growing selves.

Smoothie

I make this the night before when I'm cleaning the kitchen after dinner, and just shake it in the bottle when I'm ready to drink it in the morning. The recipe below makes a large serve, so I have half at home, and the rest as a late brekky/morning tea around 9 am in the practice.

- 30 g of protein*

- 100 g of frozen blueberries

- 100 mL of milk of choice (I use rice milk)

- approx. 400 mL of water

Mix well in a blender or Thermomix.

Other ingredients we sometimes add:

- different fruits (banana, mango, dragonfruit)

- spinach leaves

- nut butter

- ice (makes it like a thickshake)

- kids' vitamin C (I use Nutraorganics berry powder if my kids need an immune boost).

Boiled eggs and toast

This one isn't rocket science. Each egg is about 10 g of protein. As a mum, if you can get 30 g of protein in your brekky you will feel full and your cells will love you. With the kids, I aim for about 20 g, since they are smaller.

---

*You can use collagen powder or neutral-flavoured whey proteins. If you're sharing with the kids, be mindful that some of the 'work-out' powders have added extras that might not be suitable for kids.

The toast will fill them up. Add some avocado on the side for some healthy fats and good brain food for both you and them. Voilà, a super balanced brekky.

Eggs in tomatoes

www.foodandwine.com/recipes/mexican-eggs-baked-in-tomato-sauce

This is one of my weekend favourites. It takes some time (there is no chance I will do this during the week), but if I'm feeling like a slow and delicious start to the day it works a treat.

The kids eat it without the chilli, and with the eggs on toast. It's super delish and healthy for you too!

Smoothie bowl

minimalistbaker.com/super-green-smoothie-bowl

I have to admit I rarely make this, but a few of my mama friends find this a great way to get fruit into their kids and they sneak collagen and vitamin C powder in for them too, to up the protein stakes.

Homemade granola

wholefoodsimply.com/granola-toasted-muesli

When we were into Paleo, I used to make this granola each weekend in preparation for the week. We would have it with coconut yoghurt. Now, it's more of a holiday treat, and I make it with Greek yoghurt, honey and fresh fruit. We still love it, and we often make a double batch so it lasts forever.

Matilda's salad plate

Yep...my daughter digs salad for brekky. Weird, but I'm not complaining because it's pretty healthy. She loves cut-up cucumber, carrot, ham and occasionally avocado. I'll often sneak in a side serve of scrambled eggs.

When making scrambled eggs, I literally use eggs with nothing added. No milk, no cheese. I cook them for about 30 seconds in a pan on the stove top. Simple!

Our family Korean brekky

When we lived in South Korea, I had all the time in the world to make luscious brekky feasts. But this one was super quick, and even the kids (when they were little) would eat it. It still gets whipped out during winter or if we need a warm hug. It's a poached egg and broth soup with veggies.

1. Have 1 to 1.5 cups of broth* per person bubbling away in a pan.

2. Stir through some greens (I love silverbeet, the kids dig spinach).

3. Poach some eggs in the broth. Just crack them in when it's simmering and they will kinda stick together. And that's it!

4. I add chilli sauce on top. The kids definitely don't.

---

* You can slow cook the broth. These days you can even get organic broth from the supermarkets in the gravy section or fridge. If you want to make it yourself, here's my fave broth recipe: www.quirkycooking.com. au/2014/05/bone-broths-meat-stocks

Celery juice

This is pretty self-explanatory. Lots of people swear by this as a cleansing aide and to help your system reset or detox. According to the website Medical Medium, celery juice is the way to go (though I'm still not sure on it all). I use it for a few days at a time if my system needs a clean out and that pure feeling.

All you do is juice celery. If you don't have a juicer, you can blend it fast and strain off the chunks.

Lunch

Easy Mama lunch 101

The easiest and most reproducible thing I do to keep my lunch healthy and nourishing is to make it the night before while I'm prepping dinner. I particularly need to do this for days I'm home all day, because otherwise I'll be reaching for foods that don't serve me so well nutritionally (I do love a frozen gluten-free meat pie—so gross but so reminiscent of my childhood).

- 1 cup of salad greens
- cucumber
- alfalfa sprouts
- bean sprouts
- 2 radishes cut up small
- 5–10 olives
- pre-roasted leftover beetroot or tinned beetroot
- 1 tbsp flaxseed oil
- 1 tsp balsamic vinegar
- ½ cup left-over roast veggies (if I have them)
- salt and pepper

Toss all the ingredients together and add a protein if you want to. When I'm planning dinner, I always cook extra to go in my and my husband's lunchboxes the next day. Proteins that I sometimes add include:

- Cajun chicken breast

- steak

- turkey rissoles

- drumsticks

- fish

- butterflied lamb roast

- Peking duck breasts (from the supermarket—so good if you haven't tried them, and easy too)

Just as with brekky, I try really hard to get a decent amount of protein in. It fills me up, and gives me the get-up-and-go to keep on going. I also find that when I'm busy in my practice in the afternoon, a carrot (and a small serve of cheese/nuts or similar) mid arvo and a herbal tea is enough for me if I've had a decent serving of protein at lunchtime.

Cajun lemon lime chicken

This is a really easy recipe. You can change the spice up for whatever you want, and just add and subtract chicken and juice according to the number of mouths you have to feed.

- 2 chicken breasts, sliced into 3 big pieces

- juice of a lemon

- juice of a lime

- 2 tbsp of Cajun/Moroccan/taco/Italian herbs

- 2 tbsp of olive oil

I'd like to say I marinate the chicken, but I generally don't. I just lather it in all the spices by shaking it in a ziplock bag, and then pop the oil in the pan and start cooking. I use the lemon and lime juice in the cooking process by pouring it on and around the chicken if I didn't marinate it. If I did, I just tip all of the juice in with the chicken.

This can also easily be dinner. We serve it with sweet potato chips and coleslaw or mash and veggies.

Quiche/frittata

Because I am a coeliac, you will notice a lot of the dishes I share have no gluten in them. I began making crustless quiches to fill up hungry lunchboxes, and also to use up leftovers. I have used a chickpea crust on my quiche in the past (I'll pop the link below). Some day-care/school facilities are okay with eggs; others aren't. So make sure you check the deets before you swing it into lunchboxes.

- This one has four different versions of filling: www.australianeggs.org.au/recipes-and-cooking/quiche-four-ways
- This is an awesome Quiche Lorraine that I love: www.recipetineats.com/quiche-lorraine
- This is my go-to frittata recipe: cookieandkate.com/best-frittata-recipe
- And here is the chickpea crust for those of you with the same dilemma as me: www.queenofmykitchen.com/classic-quiche-with-a-chickpea-flour-crust/#recipejump

Sausage rolls

These are a simple throw-together that I hide veggies in for the kids. They fill up lunchboxes nicely. My grandma would be mortified, but I use frozen puff pastry for these—either GF or normal—and it works a treat.

For this recipe I use my Thermomix, but I will chat you through puff pastry how I would do it non-Thermie too.

I make a huge batch and freeze them for lunchboxes.

- puff pastry (approximately 3 sheets for 500 g mince)
- beef and pork/veal mince (500 g in total)

Blend together the minces. (You can use any mince really. I've made these with turkey mince too, but they are a bit dry.)

- 1 onion and some garlic, cut up and cooked off slightly to soften the onion
- 2 eggs
- 1 big squirt of tomato sauce
- 1 big squirt of BBQ sauce
- 1 grated carrot
- 1 grated zucchini

Blend all of these ingredients together.

Slightly roll out the puff pastry. Cut each sheet in half. Place a small amount of the filling on each half of the puff pastry (approx. 2.5 cm from the front edge). Roll front to back until the seam is underneath. Place them on a baking tray. Cut short slits into the pastry, and wash with some milk or egg. Repeat until all the filling is used up.

Cook at 180° C for about 20 minutes for non GF and about 35 minutes for GF.

Meatballs

I often cook up meatballs without sauce and add these to the kids' lunchboxes. Like you, I don't have heaps of time to make meatballs, so I get the prepared ones from the supermarket and fry them. A great non-sandwich alternative for lunchboxes or protein for salads. If you want a recipe, here's one I think looks pretty good:

www.tasteofhome.com/recipes/quick-and-simple-meatballs

Pizza scrolls

www.thermobexta.com.au/2014/11/09/spelt-scrolls-sweet-or-savoury

Again, I keep this easy. (I could make dough in my Thermomix.) Here's a spelt recipe that you could use . . . but I'm often not into making dough rise unless I'm on holidays or have plenty of time. Also, in this recipe I would forego the spelt grain and just use that amount in spelt flour—because we are mums and that is easier 😊

But for the cheat's version, again I use puff pastry from the freezer. Let it thaw. Slightly roll it so it's a bit bendy. Then I use pizza sauce, ham and cheese. Or I use Vegemite and cheese. And just once I've done jam with a bit of cinnamon.

They aren't super fat and puffy if you use GF pastry, but they do give the kids a crunchy yummy to have in their lunchboxes, and they're quick and easy to make.

Homemade sushi

www.fifteenspatulas.com/homemade-sushi

This is something the kids love to do with me. I was always scared of this, but it's actually pretty easy and fun, and the mess isn't too extreme. We use avocado and canned tuna generally, occasionally with some grated carrot. But the great thing is, you can make anything taste good in them.

Dinner

I don't know about you, but dinner is often the trickiest with kids. They want something, you want something else ... and then they don't eat what you have cooked anyway.

I thought I would bring together some of the simple recipes that I have used over the years. To keep it real though, on time-poor nights I do stick a lot with simple mash and veggies and a protein.

Mash

We generally use sweet potato/pumpkin/carrots. I find that too much white potato makes me feel slow. Yummy.

Baked veggies

My kids are pretty used to my wild baked veggies. I often sprinkle them with oil, dukkha, salt or herbs. I always cook an extra tray of veggies. Some go in salads, some are used on Tuesday nights to heat up for leftovers when I'm at work late. Some regular varieties include:

- parsnip
- zucchini
- beetroot
- sweet potato
- potato
- carrot
- steamed veggies.

Pretty self-explanatory. I steam carrots, beans, broccoli, zucchini and corn as a general rule and then add in the baked veggies or mash as well.

If we are having an Asian-inspired protein, I sprinkle some sesame oil on when they are finished. Otherwise, we leave it simple.

Sauteed veggies

A lot of the week I crave extra greens at night, so I cut up what I have — generally some kale, silverbeet, asparagus, broccolini and cabbage — and sauté them all. The kids will not eat this, but I do keep offering it to them. Hopefully one day they will change their mind.

To do this, I melt a small amount of butter/ghee and a dash of olive oil. Pop in some garlic, then add in the greens. Once they're cooked and soaked up the oil, I add in ¼ cup of water or broth and let them simmer down. Towards the end I'll add in a sprinkle of soy sauce, tamari or sesame oil. I also often add in nutritional yeast (great for B12).

Protein

All of these options are easy to make extra to go in lunches the next day, decreasing the load in your day!

You've seen my Cajun chicken in the lunch section. It gets trotted out at least once a month.

I find the protein part pretty easy. This is easily my go-to during the week. I can get the veggies in, mash boiling in water, steamer tray on top and protein cooking in a pan and on the table in 25 minutes — great for busy nights after sport.

- steak (the kids will eat it, or sometimes I cook them sausages instead)
- lamb chops
- sausages

- Peking duck pre-cooked in the fridge at the supermarket that I just heat up in the oven. Then I use the Peking sauce on the veggies too. I also use this with noodles.

- chicken strips, crumbed and cooked off

- rissoles

- pork chops

- salmon

- fish, crumbed in either GF breadcrumbs or almond meal. I do a layer of tapioca/potato starch, egg, then the crumb. Goes down a treat.

My fave... the gluten free version of KFC. I make this for special nights like footy: glutenfreeonashoestring.com/gluten-free-fried-chicken-kfc-style

Homemade burgers

I buy burger buns, cut up some sweet potato into chip shapes and make homemade burgers often. They are delish!

Here is a recipe if you need help:

www.taste.com.au/recipes/homemade-beef-burger/cb9272c2-d862-428f-b807-1507b84fdbd6

I will sometimes also use the frozen beetroot patties that you get at the supermarket if we are trying for a meat-free protein.

And I have also changed up the buns for either cos lettuce leaves or baked mushrooms.

So many choices.

Tacos

Great with kids because they can build their own. Trust me ... these are a taste sensation and they take about 30 minutes all up!

I also love a soft taco with:

- caramelised onion (I make this, but do it for a max. of 10 minutes—not as sweet, but still great. www.taste.com.au/recipes/caramelised-onions/5e9306e9-8c70-48dc-98ea-d1f646b6065d)

- haloumi strips cooked off

- cucumber strips

- mayo

- roasted sweet potato chips.

Japchae (Korean glass noodle stir fry)

drivemehungry.com/japchae-korean-glass-noodles

The kids love this, and it's the only way I can get stir fry into anyone else in my house. I find the sweet potato glass noodles in the Asian section of most supermarkets now, and it reminds us of living in South Korea.

It always makes a lot so there's leftovers for lunch.

Mexican lasagne

simplygluten-free.com/blog/2013/05/gluten-free-mexican-lasagna-recipe.html

If I'm making dinner at lunchtime, this is one that we like and can easily be gluten free as well. A different take on normal lasagne, but definitely worth a try.

Slow cooker ribs

cafedelites.com/slow-cooker-barbecue-ribs/

A simple set-and-forget option if I'm busy in the day is ribs. I buy them from the butcher when they are on special. Easy and delish!

I literally throw them in the slow cooker, rub them with a spice mix for BBQ (smoky chipotle or something). Throw in at least a cup of pureed tomatoes and a cup of beef stock, and let them go for the day.

When I get home, I transfer them to a baking tray. Sometimes I will pop some BBQ Texan sauce on top, and bake them for 20 minutes to give them a little crunch.

Serve with veggies and/or salad.

Slow cooker honey chicken

www.taste.com.au/recipes/slow-cooker-honey-garlic-chicken-recipe/ ggkt7bgo

Occasionally I will add some steamed broccoli on the side so I feel less guilty about the lack of veggies, but I must admit it's a great cook for lunch or dinner.

This also goes well with rice and the sauce dripped into it for leftover kids' food for a few days after. I did this with plenty of my recipes when the kids were little.

Skinnymixers pork belly

skinnymixers.com.au/skinnymixers-roast-pork-belly-with-caramelised-apple-sauce

My fave dinner whether I have had an amazing day or a shit one. This is a Thermomix recipe. (So sorry for the non-Thermies out there.) But if you are chasing caramelised apple sauce and twice cooked pork belly, then this is for you. The kids will eat the pork, but the crackling only minimally!

I hope these ideas can spark up your food selections a bit more! I know that just learning that the meat-and-three-veg option, while often a bit boring, is really the easiest way to feed the family was a lifesaver for me. Changing up the protein, or grabbing a bag of pre-done salad from the supermarket, makes the kids feel like they are getting something different, when really it's all pretty similar.

I haven't popped in a lot of staples. I am sure you have a handle on meals like spag bol. We love that in our house, as I'm sure you do.

Happy nourishing yourself and your fambam!

Ali

REFERENCES

Introduction

Azhari, A., Leck, W. Q., Gabrieli, G., Bizzego, A., Rigo, P., Setoh, P., Bornstein, M. H., Esposito, G. (2019). Parenting stress undermines mother-child brain-to-brain synchrony: a hyperscanning study. *Scientific Reports 9*, 11407. Doi: 10.1038/s41598-019-47810-4

Chapter 2

BabyCenter (n.d.). The new-mom body survey: 7,000 women tell it like it is. www.babycenter.com/baby/postpartum-health/the-new-mom-body-survey-7-000-women-tell-it-like-it-is_3653252

Center on the Developing Child. (2007). *In brief: the science of early childhood development*. Harvard University. https://developingchild.harvard.edu/resources/inbrief-science-of-ecd/

Dworkin S. L., Wachs F. L. (2004) 'Getting your body back': Postindustrial fit motherhood in *Shape Fit Pregnancy* Magazine. *Gender and Society*, *18*(5), 610–24. www.jstor.org/stable/4149421

Harwood, K., McLean, N., Durkin, K. (2007). First-time mothers' expectations of parenthood: What happens when optimistic expectations are not matched by later experiences? *Developmental Psychology*, *43*, 1–12. Doi: 10.1037/0012-1649.43.1.1

Lazarus, K., Rossouw, P. J. (2015). Mothers' expectations of parenthood: The impact of pre-natal expectations on self-esteem, depression, anxiety, and stress post birth. *International Journal of Neuropsychotherapy*, *3*(2), 102–23. Doi: 10.12744/ijnpt.2015.0102-0123

Madden, V., Domoney, J., Aumayer, K., Sethna, V., Iles, J., Hubbard, I., Giannakakis, A., Psychogiou, L., Ramchandani, P. (2015). Intergenerational transmission of parenting: Findings from a UK longitudinal study. *European Journal of Public Health*, *25*(6), 1030–5. Doi: 10.1093/eurpub/ckv093

Mikolajczak, M., Roskam, I. (2020). Parental burnout: Moving the focus from children to parents. *New Directions for Child and Adolescent Development*, *174*, 7–13. https://doi.org/10.1002/cad.20376

Schaffner, A. K. (2021). Living with your inner critic: 8 helpful worksheets and activities. 26 August. https://positivepsychology.com/inner-critic-worksheets

Chapter 3

Athan, Aurélie: www.matrescence.com

Buckley S. J. (2015). Executive summary of hormonal physiology of childbearing: Evidence and implications for women, babies, and maternity care. *Journal of Perinatal Education*, *24*(3), 145–53. Doi: 10.1891/1058-1243.24.3.145

East, L. (2019). Matrescence: Why mothers are feeling lost and confused. More to Mum: www.moretomum.com.au/2019/08/19/matressence

Glaser, E. (2021). Parent trap: Why the cult of the perfect mother has to end. *The Guardian.* 18 May. www.theguardian.com/lifeandstyle/2021/may/18/parent-trap-why-the-cult-of-the-perfect-mother-has-to-end

Kabbaz, A. T. (2019). *Mama rising: Discovering the new you through motherhood.* Hay House.

Sullivan, C. (2014). Bad mum guilt: The representation of 'work-life balance' in UK women's magazines. *Community Work & Family*, *18*(3), 284–98. Doi: 10.1080/13668803.2014.970128

Chapter 4

Breit, S., Kupferberg, A., Rogler, G., Hasler, G. (2018). Vagus Nerve as modulator of the brain-gut axis in psychiatric and inflammatory disorders. *Front Psychiatry*, *9*(44). www.ncbi.nlm.nih.gov/pmc/articles/PMC5859128

Cherry K., Lakhan S. (2021). How experience changes brain plasticity. VeryWellMind, Biological Psychology. www.verywellmind.com/what-is-brain-plasticity-2794886

Doidge, N. (2010). *The brain that changes itself*. Scribe Publications.

Fayaz, I. (2016). *How dehydration affects your brain*. The Brain & Spine Institute of North Houston. 16 February. https://fayazneurosurgery.com/how-dehydration-affects-your-brain/

McKay, S. (2018). *The women's brain book: The neuroscience of health, hormones and happiness*. Hachette, pp. 185–216.

Mualem R., Leisman, G., Zbedat, Y., Ganem, S., Mualem, O., Amaria, M., Kozle, A., Khayat-Moughrabi, S., Ornai, A (2018) The effect of movement on cognitive performance. *Frontiers in Public Health*. 20 April. www.frontiersin.org/articles/10.3389/fpubh.2018.00100/full#B1

Pillay, S. (2016). How simply moving benefits your mental health. Harvard Health Publishing, Harvard Medical School, 28 March. www.health.harvard.edu/blog/how-simply-moving-benefits-your-mental-health-201603289350

Ratey, J. J., Loehr, J. E. (2011). The positive impact of physical activity on cognition during adulthood: A review of underlying mechanisms, evidence and recommendations. *Reviews in the Neurosciences*, *22*(2), 171–85. https://pubmed.ncbi.nlm.nih.gov/21417955

Sacks, O. (2011). *The man who mistook his wife for a hat*. Pan MacMillan.

Todd, W. (2016). Achieve greater health by learning to balance your physical, chemical and emotional wellbeing. SD Protocol. www .sdprotocol.com

Todd, W. (2016). *SD Protocol*. Book Baby.

Voytek, B. (2013). Brain metrics: How measuring brain biology can explain the phenomena of mind. *Scitable* by Nature Education, 20 May. www.nature.com/scitable/blog/brain-metrics/are_there_really_as_many

Weaver, L. (2017) *Rushing women's syndrome: The impact of a never ending to-do list on your health*. Little Green Frog Publishing.

Chapter 5

AIFS (Australian Institute of Family Studies). (2016). Work and family. https://aifs.gov.au/facts-and-figures/work-and-family

AIS (American Institute of Stress). (n.d.) What is stress? www.stress.org/ daily-life

The American Institute of Stress (AIS). www.stress.org/daily-life

Berthelon, M., Kruger, D., Sanchez, R. (2018) Maternal stress during pregnancy and early childhood development. IZA Institute of Labor Economics, April. https://ftp.iza.org/dp11452.pdf

Center for Substance Abuse Treatment (US). (2014). Trauma-informed care in behavioral health services. Rockville (MD): Substance abuse and mental health services administration (US). (Treatment Improvement Protocol (TIP) Series, No. 57.) www.ncbi.nlm.nih.gov/ books/NBK207201

Dispenza, J. (2012). *Breaking the habit of being yourself*. Hay House.

Evans, A., Coccoma, P. (2017). *Trauma-informed care: How neuroscience influences practice*. Routledge.

Godin, S. (2008) *Tribes: We need you to lead us*. Portfolio.

PANDA (Perinatal Anxiety & Depression Australia). (2019) Caring for someone with perinatal anxiety and depression. www.panda.org.au/health-professionals/health-professionals-resource-hub

World Health Organization (WHO). (2019). Burnout an 'occupational phenomenon': International Classification of Diseases. www.who.int/news/item/28-05-2019-burn-out-an-occupational-phenomenon-international-classification-of-diseases

Chapter 6

Dahlen, H. G., Thornton, C., Fowler, C., Mills, R., O'Loughlin, G., Smit, J., Scmied, V. (2019). Characteristics and changes in characteristics of women and babies admitted to residential parenting services in New South Wales, Australia in the first year following birth: A population-based data linkage study 2000–2012. *BMJ Open*, *9*(9), e030133. Doi: 10.1136/bmjopen-2019-030133

Kesberg, R., Keller, J. (2018). The relation between human values and perceived situation characteristics in everyday life. *Frontiers in Psychology, 9*. Doi: 10.3389/fpsyg.2018.01676

Mineo, L. (2017). Good genes are nice, but joy is better. *The Harvard Gazette.* https://news.harvard.edu/gazette/story/2017/04/over-nearly-80-years-harvard-study-has-been-showing-how-to-live-a-healthy-and-happy-life

Chapter 7

Better Health Channel. 'Protein'. Victorian Government. www.betterhealth.vic.gov.au/health/HealthyLiving/protein#protein-foods

Crosby, L. 'The carbohydrate advantage'. Physicians Committee for Responsible Medicine. www.pcrm.org/good-nutrition/nutrition-information/the-carbohydrate-advantage

Fritsche, K. L. (2015). The science of fatty acids and inflammation. *Advances in Nutrition*, *6*(3), 293S–301S. Doi: 10.3945/an.114.006940

Hibbeln, J. R., Nieminen, L. R., Blasbalg, T. L., Riggs, J. A., Lands, W. E. (2006). Healthy intakes of n−3 and n−6 fatty acids: estimations considering worldwide diversity. *The American Journal of Clinical Nutrition*, *83*(6), 1483S–93S. Doi: 10.1093/ajcn/83.6.1483S.

Joseph, M. (2018). '27 whole food sources of fat that are rich in nutrients'. Nutrition Advance. www.nutritionadvance.com/low-carb-whole-food-fat-sources

Simopoulos, A. P. (2016). An increase in the omega-6/omega-3 fatty acid ratio increases the risk for obesity. *Nutrients*, *8*(3), 128. Doi: 10.3390/nu8030128.

Chapter 8

Brooks, K., Carter J. (2013) Overtraining, exercise and adrenal insufficiency. *Journal of Novel Physiotherapies*, *3*(125). https://pubmed.ncbi.nlm.nih.gov/23667795/

Dugan, S. A., Frontera, W. R. (2000). Muscle fatigue and muscle injury. *Physical Medicine and Rehabilitation Clinics of North America*, *11*(2), 385–403. Doi: 10.1016/S1047-9651(18)30135-9

McGonigal, K. (2020). Five surprising ways exercise changes your brain. *Greater Good Magazine.* https://greatergood.berkeley.edu/article/item/five_surprising_ways_exercise_changes_your_brain

Physiotherapy in Motion. (2021) Five facts about…female pelvic health. https://australian.physio/inmotion/five-facts-about-…-female-pelvic-health

Szumilewicz, A., Dornowski, M., Piernicka, M., Worska, A., Kuchta, A., Kortas, J., Błudnicka, M., Radzimiński, Ł., Jastrzębski, Z. (2019). High-low impact exercise program including pelvic floor muscle exercises improves pelvic floor muscle function in healthy pregnant women: A randomized control trial. *Front Physiol.*, *9*, 1867. Doi: 10.3389/fphys.2018.01867.

Chapter 9

Bhavanani, A.B., Ramanathan, M., Madanmohan. (2014). Immediate effect of alternate nostril breathing on cardiovascular paramaters and reaction time. *Online International Interdisciplinary Research Journal.* http://icyer.com/documents/ANB_CYTER_2014.pdf

Vogel, K. (2020). Brené Brown's 3-Step Approach to Transcending Failure and 'Rising Strong'. *Maybe It's Just Me.* https://maybeitsjustme. blog/2019/02/28/brene-browns-3-step-approach-to-transcending-failure-and-rising-strong/amp/

Mayo Clinic. (2020). Positive thinking: Stop negative self-talk to reduce stress. www.mayoclinic.org/healthy-lifestyle/stress-management/in-depth/positive-thinking/art-20043950

Moore, C. (2021). Positive daily affirmations: Is there science behind it? Positive Psychology. https://positivepsychology.com/daily-affirmations/

Raghuraj P., Telles S. (2008). Immediate effect of specific nostril manipulating yoga breathing practices on autonomic and respiratory variables. *Applied Psychophysiology and Biofeedback, 33*(2), 65–75. Doi: 10.1007/s10484-008-9055-0.

Chapter 10

Chek, Paul. (n.d.). Managing sleep challenges. The Chek Institute: https://chekinstitute.com/blog/managing-sleep-challenges

National Institute on Aging. (2020). A good night's sleep. US Department of Health & Human Services. www.nia.nih.gov/health/good-nights-sleep

PANDA. (n.d.). How are you sleeping? www.panda.org.au/info-support/after-birth/how-are-you-sleeping

Suni, E. (2021). Sleep deprivation. Sleep Foundation. www.sleepfoundation.org/sleep-deprivation

Yang, Y., Li, W., Ma, T-J., Zhang, L., Hall, B. J., Ungvari, G. S., Xiang, Y-T. (2020). Prevalence of poor sleep quality in perinatal and postnatal women: A comprehensive meta-analysis of observational studies. *Frontiers in Psychiatry*, 13 March. www.frontiersin.org/articles/10.3389/fpsyt.2020.00161/full

Chapter 12

Lieberman, M. (2013). *Social: Why our brains are wired to connect*, Crown.

Nuss-Warren, D. (2020). Science says that cave-women were working mothers, too. *Moms*. www.moms.com/science-says-cavewomen-working-mothers/

Chapter 13

Brown, B. (2015). Own our history. Change the story. https://brenebrown.com/blog/2015/06/18/own-our-history-change-the-story/

Salters-Pedneault, K. (2020). Learning to observe and accept your emotions. verywellmind website. www.verywellmind.com/emotional-acceptance-exercise-observing-your-emotions-425373

Chapter 14

Ackerman, C. E. (2021). What is self-worth and how do we increase it? https://positivepsychology.com/self-worth

Covington, M. V., Beery, R. G. (1976). *Self-worth and school learning*. Holt, Rinehart & Winston.

Wong, S. J. (2021). 13 things that don't determine your self-worth. *Shine*. https://advice.theshineapp.com/articles/12-things-that-dont-determine-your-self-worth

Chapter 15

Fabrizio, K. (2018). Understanding maternal covert narcissism: When mom can't let go. *GoodTherapy*. www.goodtherapy.org/blog/understanding-maternal-covert-narcissism-when-mom-cant-let-go-0309185

Green, A., Charles, K. (2019) Voicing the victims of narcissistic partners: A qualitative analysis of responses to narcissistic injury and self-esteem regulation. *SAGE Open*. https://journals.sagepub.com/doi/pdf/10.1177/2158244019846693

Kaufman, S. B. (2017). Narcissism and self-esteem are very different. *Scientific American*. https://blogs.scientificamerican.com/beautiful-minds/narcissism-and-self-esteem-are-very-different/

Lancer, D. (2018). Daughters of narcissistic mothers. *Psychology Today*. www.psychologytoday.com/au/blog/toxic-relationships/201802/daughters-narcissistic-mothers

INDEX

Printed and bound by CPI Group (UK) Ltd, Croydon, CR0 4YY
14/03/2022

03116660-0001

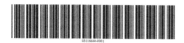